ALZHEIMER'S DISEASE

Elizabeth Forsythe qualified as a doctor in
1950 and took up writing part-time while
bringing up her family. She has recently
retired from practice to write full-time.

Dr Forsythe is the author of *Living with
Multiple Sclerosis* (1979) and *Multiple
Sclerosis: Exploring Sickness and Health*
(1988), both published by Faber and based
on her experiences as an M S patient. She
is the editor of the *British Journal of Family
Planning* and the *Faber Pocket Medical
Dictionary*.

Alzheimer's Disease
The Long Bereavement

Elizabeth Forsythe MRCS, LRCP, DPH

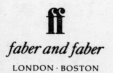

faber and faber

LONDON · BOSTON

First published in 1990
by Faber and Faber Limited
3 Queen Square London WCIN 3AU
Reprinted 1991

Photoset by Wilmaset Birkenhead Wirral
Printed in England by Clays Ltd, St Ives plc

© Elizabeth Forsythe, 1990

Elizabeth Forsythe is hereby identified as
author of this work in accordance with
Section 77 of the Copyright, Designs and
Patents Act 1988

A CIP record for this book is
available from the British Library

ISBN 0–571–14110–2

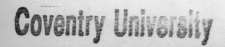

Contents

Foreword

In this accessibly written book Dr Elizabeth Forsythe tackles the problems and fears aroused by Alzheimer's disease. In her subtitle, 'The Long Bereavement', she indicates the need for multidisciplinary understanding, skill and care. As the proportion of those in the population who are aged slowly increases, so it becomes more crucial that mental diseases, including Alzheimer's, should be understood by us all, not merely relegated to the margins of everyday knowledge. Dementia is so frightening for the patient, the relatives and even at times for professional carers that this objective and sensitive treatment could not be more welcome.

The slow change of someone close to you can be very threatening. It's not only that you can't foresee how things will be with them next Christmas. You cannot even recall the past with them: it becomes impossible even to look through the family photo album or to gossip about the old days when the children were young, or that holiday you went on, or community task you did together. You grieve; you feel as if your loved one were disintegrating; your security is threatened, and you regret 'all the things left undone that we ought to have done'.

Alzheimer's disease is still not fully understood or discussed openly. Many sufferers do not ask for help because there is no cure. But many carers can be helped to make the slow goodbye that is so painful. It is painful because we rage against the tearing apart which death brings. Our own dis-eases and fears, inadequacies and sins are caught up in the gradualness of this bereavement and we lose touch with ourselves, both our health and our character.

This book will be welcomed not only by professionally concerned doctors, lawyers and carers, but by relatives and friends. Our need for common-sense, objectivity and wisdom is never greater than when caring requires so much resilience and patience. Hopelessness and sheer tiredness can take a grim grip on our resources.

Here we are given a privileged glimpse into the catharsis of pain. The strain resulting from caring, 'nerves', sleeplessness and stress within marriage and within child/parent relationships can be overwhelming, and we may find we are 'distancing' ourselves from the sufferer just in order to survive. Dr Forsythe's book offers help on how not to run away and at the same time to realize how much support we need if we are to be effective carers.

Our community, as represented by the NHS, may also be tempted to 'distance' itself from this most taxing form of care: the creation of psychogeriatric teams is expensive and still very slow. Dementia requires all types of resources, medical, personal and spiritual. Too often patients and carers have been left in a wilderness of isolation – like the biblical model of the scapegoat.

In 1990 the Church of England's Board for Social Responsibility is publishing a report on ageing, including the care of those suffering from Alzheimer's disease. Dr Forsythe gives testimony in her final chapter to our need for spiritual resources in caring for Alzheimer's disease patients. To quote another Norwich doctor, Sir Thomas Browne, of 300 years ago: 'Surely there is a piece of divinity in us, something which was before the elements and owes no allegiance to the sun.' This book will help us to face what can be a long bereavement with the faith that the Spirit will not desert us, for, as Sir Thomas Browne hinted, the Spirit is within both the victim and the carer to the very end.

Alan Webster, formerly Dean of St Paul's,
January 1990

1 / The Story of John

John was my husband and he died from Alzheimer's disease in 1986. While thinking about his life and his illness and death, I have come to see his dementia and its conclusion as a development of the sort of person he was. Increasingly it seems to me that illnesses cannot be isolated as though they are something quite separate from the people we are and John's dementia cannot be detached from the sort of person he was. I know, as a doctor, that somebody with Alzheimer's disease could not write his own story but I wonder if John could have written his own story at any time in his life, even long before the dementia started. The more I wonder, the more sure I become that he could not have. For many of us, increasing age, increasing leisure or failing physical health gives us the time and opportunity to look at our lives, to think critically about them and begin to have a clearer idea of who we are, what our lives have meant to us and those closest to us, and what their lives have meant to us. John could never have thought or talked about such things. There were large parts of his life which were always completely secret and I believe they remained hidden even from himself. In an extraordinary way his death from Alzheimer's disease was a logical end to his fragmented and hidden life.

I believe it is important to share the story of John and my understanding of the intertwining of his personality and the development of his dementia. It may help carers and others close to a dementing person to recognize more about their own problems and give them a clearer understanding of the ways in which they are able to help the dementing person as well as of the limits to such help. They may also be better able to cope with the disintegration of a person close to themselves without feeling so threatened by this terrible tragedy. I do not believe that Alzheimer's disease is a disease in the accepted sense of being some sort of illness that arrives and affects a person who was previously in good physical and mental health; but that it is a condition that develops in a person who is already at risk and has been so for many years. The difficulties in diagnosis and of management arise partly because of this subtle development. This unusual type of condition needs better understanding so that helpers can be less confused in their own minds and more ready to ask for and accept the help which they need.

John was born in 1910 and was an only child. His father, who seems to have been an outstandingly intelligent and creative man, died at the age of fifty when John was in his teens. It was extraordinary that John never spoke about his father because during the 1920s and 1930s he had been an innovative writer of mystery fiction and a talented water-colour painter. It was almost as though John preferred to deny rather than acknowledge and delight in his artistic inheritance. Possibly his father's artistic temperament contributed to the breakdown of his parents' marriage; they lived apart for a number of years during John's childhood and adolescence. I think that John was probably a shy and sensitive child and suffered during his parents' separation when he was brought up by his mother and three of her childless sisters.

His ambition had been to study engineering and he had started a course; but under pressure from family friends and with the incentive of more money and better prospects, he went into a business of city brokers. He was able, in this job, to use his considerable talents for learning, speaking and working in a variety of foreign languages. I think that he was by nature a solitary person although at times, on the surface, he seemed to enjoy being with people. During the 1939-45 war his talent for languages was of use in the secret intelligence service and his attachment to various embassies helped him develop a role of easy sociability and charm which became useful later when he returned to business life. His inner solitariness seemed to need the protection of a superficial gregariousness. By the end of his life his solitariness was uppermost and in his dementia he became totally isolated and unreachable.

When we married he was forty-five and I was seventeen years younger. To me he remained extraordinarily remote and in many ways essentially a stranger. There was an immense fascination in his remarkable talent for language and his ability to adapt to different countries and to the different roles in his life. He was a successful businessman and esteemed by his colleagues; yet there was always the sense that he was acting a role and did not see himself as a businessman. He had expensive and immaculate business suits but would then wear a shabby tweed coat over the top and a rather battered felt hat. This contradiction between the desire to be totally conventional and some secret desire to be very unconventional or even eccentric ran through all his life. He always seemed to want the appearance of one thing; but actually lived in an opposite way. He wanted the presence of a wife and the appearance of an established and 'happy' home life without the need to be committed to it. He was pleased to have children but avoided any involvement in being a father. There was always this contradictory strand of wanting to make the right appearance and to play the right role in the different spheres of his life, but at the same time avoiding the commitment that could bring reality or meaning to his relationships.

My enjoyment of closeness and warmth in relationships probably attracted him to me in the first place because these emotions had been absent in his life. These same characteristics then terrified him and our marriage became for the most part a distant relationship of varying roles. I shall never know what our relationship meant to him. Our happiest times together were while travelling either for pleasure or for his work, perhaps because we were then both equally removed from the realities of looking after a home and bringing up children and could therefore share a world on equal terms. At such times I hoped that one day these intervals of peace would be extended into what I saw as our 'real' life at home and with our family; but those hopes were never fulfilled.

He had the expatriate Scot's longing to return to his 'home-land' and in 1969 we bought some land and ruins in the far north-east of Scotland and in due course built a beautiful house overlooking a harbour and the Moray Firth. I moved up there with our three children in 1973 and John should have retired and come to live there the following year; but sadly many things happened, including changes in his firm. He did not retire until five years later, though this was apparently not his decision.

It is difficult looking back on the life of somebody who develops Alzheimer's disease to be able to say 'yes, it started at such and such a time' or even at about a certain time. This was so in John's life. But with the benefit of hindsight it is possible to see markers along the way of changes and developments in his life that point towards his final disintegration. Also with the benefit of hindsight it is easy to say that John was not at all the same person outwardly when he retired in 1978 as he was when we made the decision to move to the far north of Scotland in 1969. Looking back now, eleven years later, I am sure that in 1978 when he did retire, his 'normal' solitariness had tipped into an abnormal sort of isolation which progressed into his dementia.

Early in 1978, while John was still working in London and living in our earlier home near Cambridge, he suddenly

developed a severe pain in his back. He stayed on his own in bed
for a number of days before deciding to make the long journey
north. He arrived on the night sleeper in Inverness and was
exhausted, in a lot of pain and very depressed. He was admitted to
an orthopaedic ward in Inverness for diagnosis and treatment.
After a week he was discharged in more or less the same state and
came home to Caithness for a period of rest. Certainly he was in
pain and in great distress; but he was also, quite uncharacteristi-
cally, depressed and tearful. He did not want me out of his sight
and kept saying that he had spent all his life worrying about
possessions and ignoring people. He seemed very sad that he had
had so little time for his family during his working life and
particularly during the previous five years. He had seldom come
north and had seen remarkably little of our adolescent family.
During these weeks he slept badly and was constantly preoccupied with his feelings of sadness. He said that all he wanted now
was time to spend with me and the family and to have the
opportunity to make up for all his distance in the past. It was sad
but at the same time a moment I could see as holding great hope
for the future. At last he was going to retire and there would be
time for doing all the things together that we had talked about.
For me there was an almost unbelievable feeling of relief that all
the problems and isolation and rejection of past years might
indeed be changing. His back became less painful and he decided
to return to work in London full-time for six weeks before finally
retiring.

I shall never know whether these months prior to his return to
London were the onset of Alzheimer's disease or a depressive
illness; perhaps the distinction is unimportant. Certainly something profound and disturbing was occurring in John's mind.
Although he was depressed during the time he was at home with
his painful back, he had hopes and aspirations for his retirement
which were different from his previous way of living. For many

weeks we were extraordinarily close in sharing his sadness and both our hopes. It really did seem to be a turning point in his life and in our relationship and I felt as though a new sort of reality might be supplanting the playing of many roles. It is useless now to keep wondering if any sort of outside help could have made those possible or potential changes into a continuing reality.

I did not see John for several weeks after his return to London and when we did meet, he was once again a distant stranger and there was no more talk of spending time together. He came home to Caithness at the end of July. In 1972 he had bought an old Orkney sailing boat and had been looking forward to doing it up and sailing it. He became involved in litigation with the boatyard that was doing some of the major repairs, and it was a while before that was concluded and the boat was back in the harbour below our house and ready for him to work on. He would spend many hours getting ready to do a job on the boat so that by the time he was organized and everything was down at the harbour it was usually time for him to start clearing up again. He seemed to be constantly active and apparently occupied but in the end achieving nothing. I thought that perhaps this was another manifestation of the distress that he had shown earlier in the year and it would pass as he settled down in his retirement.

In retrospect some indication of his worsening condition might have been given by his attitude to money. John had had a substantial 'golden handshake' from his firm on his retirement. Early in 1978 during his weeks of 'depression' he had told me about the money and said that he intended to make two trusts; one to pay for the university education of our children and the other for an annuity for me because his work pension did not make provision for his widow, and with our age difference it was likely that I should outlive him. After his return to London he spoke no more about these financial provisions. When two of the children started at university in the autumn of 1978 he said that he did not have enough money to help them and did not mention his capital sum or his earlier expressed plans again. He had always been secretive about money, and I had never known what his financial position was or how much he earned. From the time of the move to Caithness I had always been short of money and did some journalism and part-time medicine to help with household bills. His sudden announcement that he was not able to make any contribution to our son and daughter's upkeep at university came as an amazing blow and I could think of no way of supporting them. He had always been mean with money. The real difference had been during the earlier months of that year, when he had wanted to be generous. It is not possible even with the benefit of hindsight to say that his dementia was now starting, because the change merged into his previous personality.

The stranger with some sense of familiarity had gone and a stranger with a chilling feel of remoteness seemed to have arrived in his place. I found myself alone, very far from relatives and friends of long standing, with somebody who apparently wished to be entirely isolated both physically and emotionally. I became full of fear, for him, for the children, for myself and for the future. At the time I saw him as an unreasonable tyrant, and I was afraid of him. John now believed that I was responsible for any problems that he had in his retirement and this was because I was English. There was nobody with whom I could discuss the whole painful situation. Had he really changed or was I different, and was there any way out of this nightmare? I could not find one, and at the end of 1980 I had a severe breakdown and went into hospital. John said that he wanted a divorce and did not want me to come home. By this time it was clear to him and probably to me that I was the one who had a 'problem' and I returned to the south on my own without job, money, home, husband, family, possessions or any understanding of what had been happening. It was a time of great confusion and it did not then occur to me that John might be mentally disturbed, because I had been so obviously mentally ill myself. It was to be a number of years before I could begin to understand that there was any need or reason to help John. Fortunately I had good friends in the south and survived.

From then on John made no contact with me. The following year he sold the house and moved to a London suburb to be near his cousin; but he did not send me any money from the sale of the house as he had previously agreed to do. However, I managed to get part-time work, rented an agricultural cottage, and the children continued at university without any financial support from John. John would not let me know his new address or his telephone number. I had no understanding of what had happened and in the end I tried not to think too much about him. I had to struggle with my own depressive illness and demanding work.

My difficulty in writing about this time even many years later does highlight some of the problems of disentangling the personality of a person from the development of dementia; and the destructive effects of a spouse's disintegration on the person nearest. I could not suddenly distance myself from John sufficiently in an emotional sense to see him objectively. He had always been in the habit of off-loading his problems on to somebody else; and I had always not only felt responsible for my own shortcomings but also been prepared to shoulder his. Neither of us had any insight into the changes that were occurring in him and having such a destructive effect on our relationship. Remarkable changes on my part would have been required to recognize the subtle differences in John which were heralding his progressing disintegration. At that time I could not have made those changes and even many years later much mental discipline is needed to do so. There is great difficulty in identifying what is normal life, that people must just get on with, and what might be some sort of illness, with which help is necessary.

Two years later our son graduated from Edinburgh University

and wanted both his parents to be at the graduation ceremony. Peter had seen John at various times and found him a bit difficult and demanding. He asked me to organize the day because he did not think that John would manage it. I had a shock when I met John that day. He looked a lot older, was very preoccupied with his poor eyesight and seemed convinced that he was going blind. (He had always had very healthy eyes.) John and I spent the afternoon together. Walking back to the hotel where I was staying I realized that he was totally preoccupied with himself. For me, these hours together had the sense of being a dream and I seemed able to enter into his world and see it as he saw it.

It was a very frightening world. John believed that he was being pestered with people demanding money from him and sending him bills for things which he had never had. I do not know if I thought that this was the truth but I took everything he said as such because it was clearly what he believed to be true at that time. I could understand that the way in which he saw the world, strange as it seemed to me, was entirely real for him. In Caithness I had felt threatened by his strange view of reality but now I was no longer dependent upon him, and the physical and emotional distance made my understanding greater.

John had no interest in what other family members were doing. I saw him that afternoon as a very sad and lonely person. I assured him that at no time would I ever ask for any financial help but that assurance did not seem to give him any relief. I also suggested that he might like to meet me sometimes in London to talk. He said that he would but he would still not allow me to have his address or telephone number. He said he would contact me.

He did not telephone me and I did not see him again for another two years; and by that time he no longer knew who I was. The meeting in Edinburgh could have been an opportunity for some sort of intervention. Sadly, I did not use it in this way to help John because I still did not recognize the real state of his mind. In any case there was nobody with whom I could have discussed the problem even if I had recognized its nature.

A year later, Peter was trying to equip a flat and asked John if he had any surplus household equipment. John said that he could take a van and meet him at the garage outside his flat. However, when Peter arrived John said that he could only give him very little because all his possessions had been stolen. Obviously this was extremely unlikely and now we know that this was part of his delusion of poverty and of being persecuted; but we failed to understand at the time and thought that he was not being very generous and possibly even a little devious. Again there was the confusion between the secretiveness of John's personality and his miserliness and the subtle change into overt delusions. It was a further sign of his retreat into a private fantasy world and a strange and what must have been a frightening life of total solitariness. Now I realize that these delusions were an essential part of his dementia.

The whole progression from being a solitary person who was always secretive about his money and never generous to his family, to the totally solitary miser who isolated himself from everybody he had known and particularly from his family, was so slow that it was quite impossible to identify the time when it was no longer 'normal' for John but some kind of disease.

The so-called 'crisis' in John's dementia, at which some sort of intervention was unavoidable, came in the summer of 1985. He was still driving his car and caused an accident. The police went to his flat to interview him but probably realized that he was not able to give evidence and finally dropped any charges against him. His driving licence was confiscated. His cousin kept in touch with me and finally wanted me to go and see him. I had not previously been to John's flat but it was immediately identifiable by all the locks, spy-holes on the door and strange signs and messages about where to put things. I could hear John walking about inside but it was about ten minutes before he came to the door. I could see him looking through one of the spy-holes and then he finally opened the door a crack while it was still chained. He did not appear to recognize me and was very suspicious. I just kept talking and eventually he let me in. It was the middle of a rather hot afternoon but all the curtains were drawn, some of the windows were shuttered and the heating was on. He was partly dressed and took me all the way through the flat to the furthest room which was his bedroom. It was blacked out, the electric lights were on and it was overpoweringly hot. The room was in a chaotic state, the bed was unmade and the sheets were filthy. He told me to sit down and indicated one of the two large director-type chairs in the room. Then he told me not to sit down but to put a towel on the seat first. He sat down and kept talking in a distracted way and looking at me with a puzzled expression but without recognition. I was appalled and could only bear to stay there by trying to think with the medical part of me. I could not believe that this sad and mad old man was really my husband and the person of whom I had been so afraid. I knew so little about this sort of illness, despite the fact I was a trained medical practitioner and had even done some psychiatry. At last I realized that his mind was dementing.

Eventually he went to a shelf, picked up a photograph of me, brought it over and thrust it at me, rather as a small child would, and told me that it was Elizabeth. I tried to explain that certainly it was a photograph of Elizabeth and that was me, his wife. He did not seem able to put these two ideas together. He said that he had to go through to the other section to cut the hairs on his face. He went off to the bathroom but kept returning to comment on the difficulties of shaving. I had the feeling that he also needed to check up that I was still there. I was amazed to see about fifteen clocks in his room but not one at the right time. There were two desks, piles of dirty papers, books and clothes. From one of the walls there was a branching column of electrical adaptors about twelve inches long with numerous side-branches, plugs and various radios, record-players, calculators and other devices attached. They were all so dirty that it did not look as though they had been used recently.

John continued to potter in and out and described the difficulties of putting on his tie. He was wearing a suit with a waistcoat and that also presented grave difficulties. I offered to help but he preferred to do it himself. We walked the short distance to his cousin's together but what two years previously had been a slow walk was now a shuffle. It was devastating.

During tea he kept up a loud childish prattle and constantly went off to collect other things. At one point he had to go back to his flat to find a book he wanted to show me. He was behaving like a child but not at all like the solitary, quiet, shy child I have heard he once was. He was being noisy, demanding and endlessly active. I wanted to do something to help sort it all out but I felt overpoweringly inadequate and confused. Here was the man whom I had feared so much and in reality he was just a sad old man acting like an anxious child.

John was obviously in need of help. His cousin was a lonely person following a series of bereavements and wanted him to stay near her in his own flat although his condition was deteriorating; but she did not want to have full responsibility for him. No one knew if he had any money so that we were not able to employ help or begin to investigate the possibility of moving him to a home. Anyway I doubt if he could have been persuaded to accept either of these possibilities. I could see no way out of the dilemma and went home feeling overwhelmed by the horror of the situation.

John had continued to go for private annual medical check-ups and always told his cousin that he was 100 per cent fit. He refused, however, to see his general practitioner. When I got home I telephoned his general practitioner to see if he could suggest any solution. At first it was impossible to speak to him. I wrote and received no answer. After many attempts to speak to him on the telephone I did at least begin to get to know his receptionist. She was most helpful, but the doctor remained elusive. John's cousin telephoned me frequently, often late at night, to say that it was impossible for her to cope and that I must do something. I was trying to think of some sort of solution but could not imagine what I should do. I did not even know how to find out whether he had any money so that at least I would know if he was really so poor or whether he was deluded about it.

This time of confusion and indecision was certainly bad for John; but it was also destructive for me, his family and his friends. Some of it could have been avoided if I had had some information or could have found out something about the nature of the dementia. I was certainly willing to help but failed to see what I could do or indeed that I could do anything of use. I was wrong about my inadequacy and when I did finally, many months later, make positive decisions I realized that there was a lot I could have done much earlier to relieve some of John's suffering. If his general practitioner had had some understanding of the condition and could have discussed it with me, it would have been helpful. Possibly he was ignorant about dementia or possibly he was not interested.

A doctor always puts the best interests of his patient first: but this would normally allow him to discuss all the problems of a dementing patient with the nearest relative. In this instance there were problems because I was not living with John and we did not have the same general practitioner. Or perhaps John's paranoia about his wife and family made it unlikely that a doctor would want to discuss him and certainly not with his wife.

Looking back, I realize that John could have been most helped by the person with the closest relationship to him, and that was still me. But at the time I would have needed a lot of support from committed and well-informed professionals. The general practitioner could have been the key person in organizing this support but he would have needed more knowledge and willingness to be involved. I needed to know that this is not a disease that required some sort of expert to treat it, but a person providing care and attention in many very practical ways. At the same time I also needed to be relieved of some of my guilt and feelings of total inadequacy. I needed to be told that I should not again exceed the limits of my own physical and emotional strength and must not push myself to the point of mental breakdown. This had happened before and had served no useful purpose.

In September 1985 I spent a few days with one of my wisest friends, whose mother had had dementia. It took me three days before I could bring myself to speak about John because I felt so distressed and guilty about the whole problem. She helped enormously by telling me, among other things, about power of attorney and the Court of Protection (see p. 76). I had still not managed to speak to John's doctor. Apart from my own judgement that his mind was disturbed, I therefore had no medical or any other professional support.

During the next three months I went down to see John as often as I could extricate myself from other problems, tried to get more information from his doctor and found out about the Court of Protection. However, I remained remarkably ignorant and confused about what I could or should do. Looking back now, three years later, I can see that my own failure to make any positive decisions at this time increased the confusion and everybody's distress.

Eventually I managed to make an appointment to see John's general practitioner. I discovered that at each medical check-up there had been comments about John's deteriorating mental state but his doctor said that as there was nothing he could do to help he had not contacted him. He was not enthusiastic about getting a psychogeriatrician to see him. Nothing was settled and the impossible tensions went on. John began wandering at night. The police brought him back to his cousin and his cousin telephoned me. I suggested that it might be better if, instead of having him back in his flat and the same situation being repeated, it could be the point at which he might be persuaded to go into a nursing home. She refused to say to anybody apart from myself that she could not cope. I went on procrastinating and agonizing and failing to resolve any problems.

I finally consulted an extremely well-informed and compassionate solicitor and started on the steps towards becoming the Receiver for John under the Court of Protection. The solicitor was the first professional person I had met who actually knew what he was doing and could bring all the relevant problems together and begin to resolve them. John's doctor had to sign a form to say that he was not capable of managing his own affairs. This he would not do and the delay ran into months. I telephoned and wrote to him but he continued to procrastinate. Surprisingly, some of the delays in helping John were caused by members of the medical profession, and that included me, and the greatest and most effective help came initially from the legal profession and from the clerks at the Court of Protection. This was and is extraordinary but I think it has a lot to do with the ignorance of the medical profession about the nature of dementia. The legal profession is perhaps better at looking at the evidence and the present situation; but it was possible that the doctors got entangled in the moral problem of whether I had left my husband and was now trying to get my hands on his money! That could have been one of the consequences of John's paranoia; but the legal profession seemed more objective.

However, the legal profession cannot act until the medical profession will commit itself to making a diagnosis and signing forms to that effect. Eventually I did persuade John's general practitioner to arrange a domiciliary visit from a psychogeriatrician.

I hoped that it might, at least, be possible to get the papers signed for the Court of Protection arrangements to go ahead. The visit took place and it was confirmed that John had some sort of dementia. The question of whether John should be sectioned and admitted to a mental hospital temporarily was discussed with the consultant but no decision was taken. I was not at this meeting because I was ill and unable to make the journey.

The situation deteriorated and it became clear that John could no longer live on his own. The consultant came back and after a visit from a social worker it was finally arranged that he should be sectioned and taken to a mental hospital. The general practitioner had finally been persuaded to sign the papers for the Court of Protection. The proceedings went ahead and I was amazed at the courtesy and endless help from my named contact at the Court of Protection. While John was in hospital I managed to get down to his flat and with the help of a social worker go through some of his things and begin to get his financial affairs in some semblance of order. We realized that he could afford to go into a comfortable nursing home. I decided that as John's cousin wanted him to be near her, we should look for a nursing home in that area. We found one which seemed to be good and comfortable. He could have a large ground-floor room with his own furniture, bathroom and door into a walled garden. It seemed to be the best solution and he was moved there.

Three weeks after John had been admitted to the nursing home, the agreed fee which I was paying rose sharply without any prior information. I was surprised and felt unease which later showed itself to be justified. I contacted the nursing home and discovered it had changed hands. A medical friend told me about a recently opened mental nursing home in Norfolk which had an excellent reputation. I went and saw it and was most impressed with the staff and the general atmosphere. The house and grounds were beautiful and although there was no single room available I arranged for John to be admitted three days later. Suddenly I knew what had to be done in John's best interests and I had a great sense of urgency. It is a pity that I had not had the confidence to make John's interests of paramount importance long before this.

I arranged for a medical agency to move him from one nursing home to the other – a considerable distance. The director thought that an ambulance might frighten John and sent his own car with two nurses, one of whom was a trained mental nurse; the other acted as driver. I went down with them. When I went into the nursing home I did not recognize John. He was totally rigid, could barely shuffle, was unable to swallow, so that his saliva was running down his face, and he was a strange sallow colour. He looked like a living corpse. It was horrifying, but I did not stop to discuss it with the staff apart from finding out what drugs he had been given. The most important thing now was to get him back to the quiet haven I had found for him in Norfolk. I wanted him near again, to see him regularly and to know that he was being well looked after. The journey took about four hours but it seemed never-ending. He was so rigid that we had to bend him quite hard to get him into the car. I sat beside him on the back seat and kept looking at him to see if he was still breathing. It was very difficult to see if he was or not. His face was expressionless and the only sign of life was the slightest flicker of his eyelids from time to time.

In previous years we had spent a lot of time in Norfolk on holiday. As we started driving through Thetford Forest I was aware of some sort of increased life in John. He did not move his head but his eyes seemed to be looking through the windows and I told him where we were and reminded him of all the previous times when we had driven along that road. We arrived at the nursing home and he was welcomed and made comfortable. He seemed to enjoy his supper. The matron was horrified by the state he was in and thought that he had probably had too many drugs.

This was later confirmed by their doctor. He had drug-induced Parkinsonism.

John lived for another six months. I think that for much of that time he was reasonably happy and at times I caught glimpses of a smile of recognition. Three years later I wish that I had abandoned every other activity and just spent as much time as possible with him during those months. I think that it is important to spend time with somebody who is dementing, for your own sake if not for theirs. It is easy to say that John did not know who I was. He was doubly incontinent, had to be fed and as long as he was well looked after it did not matter who did it. I understand now that every small thing I did for him during those last months helped me sort out my own confused feelings about him. In the simple acts of feeding him or helping him dress or just sitting and holding his hand, I could rekindle some of the love and tenderness I had once felt for him. It could have been a better beginning to understand all the irreconcilable emotions of anger, fear, pity and despair.

One problem was that he became very spiteful as he became more active. Sometimes he would do nothing but hit, punch and pinch. Obviously I found this very distressing. He did talk a little but it was almost impossible to understand anything of what he was saying although at times a few words were clear. He needed a great deal of care during the day and night and I was amazed at the skills and patience of the women in the nursing home. There was always a trained mental nurse on duty but most of the work was done by local girls and women from the surrounding villages with no particular training but with great gifts.

John's physical deterioration was very rapid during the last three months and he seemed to shrivel. He died in October 1986. Although he had not known who I was for more than a year, during his dying I know that he knew who I was, and could understand something that I wanted to say to him before we parted. His dying brought us back together again after many years of difficulty and much distress. His death was so peaceful and in a strange way made just a little sense of all the tragedies of the preceding years.

Three years later I thought that I should be able to write this book objectively and describe without emotion the life of John and myself, but that is not possible. The sadness goes on but now there is a little more understanding and with understanding comes relief. I feel now that knowledge about the disease also helps relieve the burden of all the 'what I might have done' thoughts and feelings. At the time of John's death and in the succeeding weeks there was some relief that his death had been peaceful, the family was together again, and for the last eighteen months of his life I had been able to play a small part in caring for him.

By the first anniversary of his death all the 'if onlys' were flooding back in and I began to understand more about the difficulties of recovering from the long bereavement that is Alzheimer's disease. I shall write more about my understanding of this problem and ways of enduring and recovering from such a prolonged experience in the last part of this book.

I am now more able to understand the damage that was done to John, to me, to our family and friends through ignorance about dementia and the very real problems of diagnosing it. This ignorance includes my own but also that of John's general practitioner. Knowledge about the disease would not have solved all the problems but it would have helped me to be more objective about John's problems and the help that I could and eventually did give. Ignorance perpetuated my own confusion, feelings of inadequacy, guilt and disbelief that I was capable of doing anything positive. John's disintegration was a very frightening threat to my own integrity: in accepting that this was so, has come the opportunity to understand very much more about myself and in so doing to be able to change and improve my relationships with those around me. Watching the disintegration of somebody close to you and experiencing it within yourself is painful, but in the end all the anguish need not be a waste.

2 / What Is Alzheimer's Disease?

cant spell

Alzheimer's disease is the commonest type of dementia and probably accounts for half the dementia of old age. Although it has the name 'Alzheimer's disease' it is not a straightforward illness like chickenpox. There is no causative virus which can be identified and no mode of transmission to be investigated and understood. Although there is now an increasing understanding of what happens to the brain during this mysterious condition, there is no understanding of why it happens.

Alois Alzheimer was a German professor of psychiatry who, in 1906, described a group of patients with this type of deterioration. A similar condition had already been described in 1835 and called incoherence or senile dementia. This was described as 'a forgetfulness of recent impressions, while the memory retains a comparatively firm hold of ideas laid up in the recesses from times long past'. Anybody who has spent time with a dementing person will recognize that description. Alzheimer also described *multi-infarct dementia* which is caused by deficiencies in the blood supply to the brain. This type accounts for about 20 per cent of dementia. Alzheimer's disease is sometimes abbreviated to AD, multi-infarct dementia to MID, and another type, described as senile dementia of the Alzheimer type, to SDAT.

To understand Alzheimer's disease more fully it is helpful to consider what a disease actually is.

What is meant by 'disease'?

Churchill Livingstone's *Pocket Medical Dictionary* defines disease as 'any deviation from or interruption of the normal structure and function of any part of the body. It is manifested by a characteristic set of signs and symptoms and in most instances its aetiology, pathology and prognosis is known.' Chambers' *20th Century Dictionary* defines disease as 'uneasiness (in this sense often written dis-ease): a disorder or want of health in mind or body'.

The medical definition of disease implies a condition occurring in a body or mind which has been previously healthy. Webster's *Medical Dictionary* defines health as 'the condition of an organism or one of its parts in which it performs its vital functions normally or properly: the state of being sound in body or mind'. Under the heading 'mental health' in the *Oxford Companion to the Mind* the characteristics of the mentally healthy person are described as 'the capacity to co-operate with others and sustain a close, loving relationship, and the ability to make a sensitive, critical appraisal of oneself and the world about one and to cope with the problems of living'.

I wrote earlier about John that I do not believe that at any time he could have written his own story. He was never able, in the words just quoted, to make a 'sensitive, critical appraisal of oneself and the world about one'. In this sense I do not believe that John was healthy at a particular time during the last ten years or so of his life and was then afflicted by a disease. I think that he had had a state of dis-ease for very many years which eventually made him unable to sustain any relationship or cope with any of the problems of daily living. Health might also be described in this context as a state of integration of body and mind and of the person with his environment and other people around him. Disease could be disintegration of the person's mind, and later body, and of the relationships around him.

It is tempting in this scientific age to expect simple answers about the cause, cure and prevention of any disease, including dementia. 'Disease' can be such a misleading word with its suggestion of something clearcut and well-defined. There is an implication that it will be curable, given enough scientific investigation. It also suggests that the disease is a distinct entity and separate from the person who has it. But it is obvious that this is not so with many so-called diseases including dementia. I believe that it is an integral part of the person who has it. The condition is threatening to those nearest to the patient precisely because there is no clearcut distinction between the person and the disease. It involves a disintegration of personality and the link between the normal and pathological person is blurred and variable as the disease progresses. This point is vital for carers to understand in order that they may remain as objective as possible.

A condition of old age Hts

Dementia is most commonly a disease of old age. About 2–3 per cent of those between the ages of sixty-five and seventy develop dementia as do more than 20 per cent of those over eighty years of age. Although these figures are given in medical literature they are subject to doubt because it is not possible to discover the true amount of dementia in the whole population. It will probably always remain to some extent a hidden condition. The patient will usually be unaware of the development of his disease and the problem is most likely to be brought to a doctor's attention by relatives or friends; or when the nearest carer can no longer carry the burden (see chapter 4). If there are many supportive people around the patient there may never be need to look for outside help.

There could be up to three quarters of a million people with dementia in the United Kingdom. The number of patients is increasing not because it is becoming a more common disease, but because there is an increasing number of people surviving into old age. The increased longevity of the population is partly due to advances in medical care – for instance, pneumonia, which has been described as 'the old man's friend', is now treatable. Dementia has a varying incidence world-wide, being much less common in the Third World and in Japan than in the developed countries of the West. Certainly the criteria for diagnosing it may vary but this does not seem to account for all the differences between various countries. It may be significant that the Third World has a much lower incidence even where there are relatively good facilities for recognizing it and where larger numbers of people are reaching old age. One of the differences could be the value that is put on old age in a culture such as that of Samoa (see chapter 10).

How does the disease start?

The onset of Alzheimer's disease is usually so insidious that nobody can say when it actually started. At first the problems may be attributed to the 'normal' changes of old age. Old people do become forgetful, and indeed even the not so old, and it is difficult to know when normal forgetfulness ends and pathological forgetfulness begins. Forgetfulness can become 'abnormal' for the family when the old person starts to wander off in the middle of the night and the police bring him home. Or when he disappears while the family or a group of friends is on holiday and then seems unaware that anybody should be alarmed. The previous personality of the patient may merge into the characteristics of the demented patient, making recognition of the onset of dementia difficult.

Many of those with dementia forget where they have put money or other valuables and then accuse others of having taken them.

We all tend to forget such things as we get older and increasingly absent-minded. It is easy to think that somebody else must have picked them up accidentally and put them somewhere. However, in dementia a time can come when there is no longer any doubt in the patient's mind that somebody else has removed the missing objects, and not accidentally but deliberately.

This sort of problem will probably not have a clear beginning because the patient could always have been the sort of person who blamed others for his own inadequacies. He may always have been a bit of a miser and then make the step to becoming deluded about the amount of money he has. From there a further development is definite delusions of poverty. 'I can no longer afford to buy food because I have no money' can later become 'I can no longer afford to buy any food because my family has stolen all my money.' This was the type of development of John's dementia and it is impossible for relatives to do anything about such changes. It causes immense distress to a family who find themselves unable either to understand or to defend themselves against the mistaken beliefs of an apparently healthy member. This insidious type of onset makes the recognition of the disease very difficult. The mixture of shame, loyalty and confusion can be very destructive for the carers, particularly if the nearest carer is the spouse.

Causes of Alzheimer's disease

The word 'causes' assumes that this is a disease in the normal medical model and for the moment I am assuming that it is so. The cause remains elusive in spite of frequent reports of discoveries. Probably no one cause will ever be found, but like other perplexing diseases it will be understood as a multifactorial disease. The factors may include the person's age, a genetic tendency, the patient's previous personality and very possibly environmental factors. Causes may be described as predisposing causes – which might include age and any genetic tendency – and precipitating causes – which could include toxins in the environment. Immediately, you can see the complications in attributing responsibility for the disease.

It is important to understand the difference between the cause of a disease and correlations between the disease and a variety of factors, many of which will be characteristics of the people who get the disease. For example, the person who has always been talkative may become the garrulous non-stop talker, the naturally dependent person become totally childish, and the person possessive of his money the miser. Advancing age correlates with the development of Alzheimer's disease but getting older is not the cause of the disease. We all get old but we do not all develop Alzheimer's disease.

Similarly there does seem to be some connection between the amount of aluminium we take into our bodies and the development of dementia (see p. 30), but aluminium is certainly not the single cause of the disease. If it were, we should all develop the disease because we all take in aluminium (see p. 29). It is not a straightforward cause-and-effect relationship and carers do need to beware of those who claim that it is. This type of oversimplification is unhelpful in the understanding of the disease. Its only effect seems to be to increase the distress.

Genetic factors

A great deal of research is being done in this area and events move too quickly for it to be possible to give a reliable or up-to-date account of the current state of knowledge in a book. I can only give some indications of the areas in which research is being done and it is best for the interested reader to keep in touch with the reports of original work published regularly by the Alzheimer's Disease Society (see p. 70). The original papers can then be traced through a public library: although they can be difficult to understand it is often worth making the effort. Information given in newspapers or on television or radio can be interesting but is often oversimplified so that 'answers' to the whole problem of the disease are given and later shown to be inaccurate. It is always difficult to distinguish between abnormalities which produce the various symptoms and those which actually started the whole disease process. It can be understood as the difference between 'what' has happened and 'why' it happened.

In the UK only one in 1,000 people of the general population under the age of sixty-five has Alzheimer's disease, but about one in three of patients has a first-degree relative with the same condition. This has the pattern of what is known as an autosomal dominant genetic disease and published studies of some families have made the disease look like this type of predictable inheritance – a very alarming possibility for members of a family in which the disease is known to exist. However, there could be other explanations including a common environmental factor or over-reporting of the disease where it has already been recognized. Some sort of genetic predisposition could need various environmental triggers before the disease would develop. At present it is certainly not believed that Alzheimer's disease has any predictable pattern of inheritance in a family.

The occurrence within a family could also be connected with familial types of personality or the ways in which a family reacts to stressful situations. One such form of stress is angry feelings: some families disguise or withdraw from such emotions by retreating into illness rather than acknowledging them. The environmental factor rather than the genetic would then be as strong.

Studies of twins can sometimes demonstrate whether a disease has a genetic or environmental cause and some studies have shown a greater incidence of both twins being affected in identical twins than in non-identical twins. However, this evidence is far from clearcut and there is no simple picture of a preponderance of genetic over environmental factors. In one pair of identical twins, both showing the clinical changes of dementia and after death the brain-changes typical of Alzheimer's disease, one twin died eleven years after the other. The latter had only been showing the clinical changes of the disease for two years. Clearly something apart from any genetic inheritance was at work in these twins.

There have been suggested links between Alzheimer's disease and Down's syndrome because middle-aged patients dying with this condition show changes in their brains which are indistinguishable from those of Alzheimer's disease. It is possible that all those with Down's syndrome will develop Alzheimer's disease if they live long enough. There has therefore been great interest in abnormalities on chromosome 21 which is the site of abnormality in Down's syndrome. One gene is associated with the synthesis of amyloid proteins in brain tissue. It has been postulated that the same gene might be responsible for abnormal amyloid deposits near blood vessels of the brain tissue in Down's syndrome and in familial types of Alzheimer's disease. However, it is no longer believed that the explanation is as simple as that, although it is still possible that some abnormality in the body's manufacture of amyloid proteins may play a part in the development of Alzheimer's disease. Again, we have to distinguish between what may cause the symptoms and what starts the disease.

Nerve growth factor, which is a protein involved in the transmission of nerve messages in brain tissue, may also be involved. Rats with experimentally induced lesions resembling those of Alzheimer's disease were given nerve growth factor and the deterioration was alleviated.

Mothers of people with Down's syndrome are usually of

maturer years. In one study this has been shown to be true also of mothers of patients with Alzheimer's disease; but it was not necessarily the last of the family who developed Alzheimer's disease. In another study there were conflicting results showing that there was no connection between maternal age and the later development of Alzheimer's disease. Once again the problems of finding any clearcut cause are demonstrated, and the need to remain aware of the limitations of scientific research is reinforced.

What about infective agents?

Scrapie is a neurodegenerative disease of sheep and it has been suggested that it might be connected with Alzheimer's disease. Scrapie, although an infectious disease, does not produce a fever and is caused by an infectious organism called a prion. When scrapie from sheep is inoculated into mice, similar changes to those associated with Alzheimer's disease are produced. However, it has not been possible to transmit Alzheimer's disease to animals and there is no evidence that Alzheimer's disease is transmissible from one human to another.

The possibility of a toxin

A number of toxins have been blamed at various times for causing Alzheimer's disease. Aluminium has been a front runner; but it is quite clear in spite of all the publicity, that aluminium is not the only cause of Alzheimer's disease. We all ingest aluminium every day in our food and drink because it is a common mineral; but we do not all get Alzheimer's disease. Therefore, even if aluminium should eventually be shown to be an important trigger, it is not the cause. Ideas of throwing out aluminium saucepans to prevent or cure Alzheimer's disease should be reconsidered. Patients with gastric problems continue to take medically approved remedies containing aluminium, although a confectionery company has been forced to withdraw a product containing a very small amount of the mineral. John, over many years, took regular doses of both an aluminium-containing product for indigestion and a fizzy medicine in the mornings which he believed increased his well-being and which also contained aluminium. Both are still on the market and I do not believe caused his dementia but of course could have played a small part in its development.

An article in the *Lancet* in January 1989 showed a relationship between the amount of aluminium in the drinking water of eighty-eight districts of England and Wales and the extent of Alzheimer's disease developing at ages of under seventy in those living in these areas. It was shown in this study that the risk of Alzheimer's disease was 1.5 times higher in districts where the mean aluminium concentration in drinking water was more than ten times higher than in other districts. Although this study is persuasive of a causal relationship between aluminium in drinking water and the likelihood of developing Alzheimer's disease, it does add the proviso that 'care is needed in interpretation because, as in all epidemiological surveys, the possibility exists that the relation observed is due to the operation of some unknown confounding variable.'

It may be difficult for us to understand such ideas. We prefer to have a straightforward theory of cause and effect. My spare bedroom ceiling developed large cracks a few weeks after one of my daughters went into the loft. It could be easy to conclude that her weight above the ceiling did the damage; but perhaps it only happened because she put a foot between the rather fragile lathes. The cracks might also be connected with the considerable age of the house, nearby bomb damage during the last war and dampness of the room because I had turned off the radiator in it during last winter to economize on fuel. Therefore, having considered all these 'confounding variables' I no longer conclude that my daughter's weight was the 'cause' of the cracks in my ceiling; but her weight could have been a contributory factor amongst many others.

Another way of looking at this problem is to see that a brick thrown at a window is likely to break it. The thickness of the glass will be a contributory factor, but its importance is minor in relation to the size and speed of the brick.

In January 1989, the BBC broadcast a *Horizon* programme about the inhabitants of the village Umatac on the Pacific island of Guam where senile dementia and Parkinson's disease are 100 times more common than anywhere else in the world. It was called *The Poison that Waits* and the script can be obtained from the BBC. The programme was a fascinating detective story, but perhaps its weakness was the need to find an answer before the end of the story and the programme. The possible 'cause' of this extraordinary incidence of degeneration of the nervous system may be a plant toxin in the cycad nut which the islanders grind and use in flour. If not prepared correctly it is known to be a dangerous poison.

The high incidence of dementia in Guam was first observed in 1946 and similar levels have since been recognized in isolated communities along the River Ia in New Guinea and on the Kii peninsula in Japan. These three areas have a common geological substrate and a high aluminium content in water, food and soil. The programme also showed that these communities of people all eat the cycad nut in one way or another. A confounding factor showed that those who had moved from Guam to America still had a high incidence of neurodegenerative diseases although some had not been living on Guam for many years.

This remarkable programme was a demonstration of the immense complexity of understanding a multifactorial condition. It showed how difficult it is for us to live with questions rather than demanding answers, even if incomplete. A Regular Review in the *British Medical Journal* in October 1988 gave a competent summary of the findings in the three areas being investigated in the *Horizon* programme and suggested that aluminium may play an indirect part by altering the metabolism of minerals which include calcium, magnesium and iron. It also commented on the current decline of the disease in these localized areas which may be partly due to supplements of calcium and magnesium to the inhabitant's diet. It states that

> the areas have also become increasingly Westernized and the local diet has moved away from dependence on flour made from the cycad nut ... Migrants from these areas have developed the disorders years later, suggesting that an environmental insult interacts with the ageing process leading to the disorder once a threshold has been passed.

That summary shows what a great difference there is between statements such as 'aluminium or the cycad nut causes Alzheimer's disease, motor neurone disease or Parkinson's disease', and the beginning of the much deeper and more difficult concept of a condition with multifactorial causes. Readers might find it interesting to study that review article. The reference is in the appendix: libraries would provide a photocopy.

What happens in the brain?

The work of the brain is controlled by nerve cells or neurons. These communicate with each other by dendrites which pass electrical messages to the neighbouring cells. Between the cells there is a gap, and the messages get through the gaps by using chemical substances called neurotransmitters. One neurotransmitter is acetylcholine and this is deficient in the brains of people with Alzheimer's disease. This is of interest because acetylcholine is known to be involved with memory. Unfortunately, the system which manages acetylcholine in the brain is complicated, with many unknown factors. There is as yet no way of supplying the deficient neurotransmitter although attempts have been made to do so.

During the course of the disease the brain shrinks. The surface lobes of the normal brain are convoluted and the potential gaps between them are called sulci. As the disease progresses, the lobes become less convoluted and the surface flattens. At the same time the sulci between the lobes widen. Inside the brain there are spaces, the ventricles, through which the cerebrospinal fluid circulates. These spaces expand during the disease. If the brain of a person with Alzheimer's disease is examined after death, characteristic microscopic changes are found. Senile plaques are found in both Alzheimer's disease and the ageing brain. They occur near the outside of the brain and are larger than the normal neurons which they replace. They are made up of abnormal nerve tissue. Neurofibrillary tangles are characteristic of Alzheimer's disease and are found inside the neurons. They have small amounts of aluminium at their centre. Other body cells, apart from brain cells, of patients with Alzheimer's disease may be unusually prone to damage because they have a defect in the process which uses oxygen. This could be responsible for the marked loss of weight and muscle wasting which often occurs late in the course of dementia. The patient may eat ravenously but just seem to fade away.

Multi-infarct dementia

In multi-infarct dementia, the brain deteriorates because of poor blood supply. The damage is patchy and the site depends on where there is interference with the blood supply. The patient is usually known to have high blood pressure and there may be a history of strokes and possibly epilepsy starting late in life. There may also have been repeated short spells of giddiness or loss of consciousness. These are sometimes called transient ischaemic attacks or TIAs. In multi-infarct dementia there are many small areas of deterioration with softening, called focal necrosis, in the brain and dementia may not be the first or only sign of damage. The progress of the disease is characteristically stepwise, which means times of getting worse, sometimes following a fit or TIA, and then times of seeming a bit better and remaining well for a while before the next episode.

Alzheimer-type and multi-infarct dementia can occur in the same patient so that there may be no clear distinction between the two types either during life or in the brain changes found after death.

Depression and dementia

Many old people do develop clinical depressive illnesses for which there are no obvious reasons and it can be difficult to distinguish between such a depressive illness and the onset of dementia. Sometimes during a depressive illness a person can appear to be dementing but this problem disappears after successful treatment of the depressive illness. This is sometimes described as 'pseudodementia'. It can be difficult to unravel depression and dementia and in any conflicting diagnosis it is usual to treat a suspected underlying depressive illness. It is not currently believed that depression is a cause of dementia.

Other types of dementia

The other 10 per cent of cases of dementia in old age are caused by a variety of problems and some of these are treatable. Acute infective illnesses and metabolic disorders can cause temporary dementia which is reversible when the underlying condition is treated. An acute infective illness will be treated with antibiotics.

Metabolic causes include thyroid and vitamin B12 deficiency. These can be diagnosed and given the correct replacement treatment. Long-standing syphilis causes brain damage and dementia and with treatment the condition is arrestable. In the future there will be an increasing problem with AIDS. There are also mechanical causes of brain destruction which may show as dementia; and these include brain tumours, chronic subdural haematomata and normal pressure hydrocephalus.

There are genetic causes of dementia which are as yet untreatable. These include Huntington's chorea, Pick's disease and a very rare and rapidly fatal type called Jakob-Creutzfeld disease.

3 / What Does Dementia Look Like?

There is no one typical picture of a person with dementia because there are different types of dementia. There are of course also many different types of people, and the way in which the condition develops will have an individual variation. Dementia can start at any age although onset is very rare before late middle age. The disease is called presenile dementia if it starts before the age of sixty, and senile dementia if it starts after that age. The two main types of dementia which start in later life are Alzheimer's disease and multi-infarct dementia, described in chapter 2.

These types of dementia cause an overall decline in a person's intellect, personality, memory and behaviour. In fact the whole person deteriorates, and late in the illness there may also be a marked physical decline. The start of the illness is usually very gradual so that in retrospect it is difficult to say when the change started or to pinpoint the last time when the person was truly him or herself. The person's previous personality may change so slowly and subtly that it merges gradually into the patient with dementia.

This is not the same as the normal deterioration which affects most people as they get old. Our brains are physically at their most effective when we are in our twenties and from that time there is a slight but continuous deterioration. However, for most people such a loss of brain power will not become too great a handicap. Names of people may be forgotten and increasing 'absent-mindedness' can be a nuisance – for example, constantly mislaid reading glasses. Dementia is caused by physical changes in the brain which are more than, and different from, the pathological effects of 'normal' ageing. Dementia needs to be clearly distinguished from ageing. If we live to be very old we do not automatically develop dementia, although our chances of developing some form of it do increase if we live to be over eighty.

It is difficult to estimate how many people of any particular age have dementia. It is not a problem that families talk about and it is easy to say that a relative is 'old' and is therefore failing mentally. As long as there is a spouse, a member of the family or friend to cope with all the problems and care for the person, it may never be recognized that he or she is suffering from dementia. The 'patient' concerned will certainly not go to a general practitioner to complain about it. The family may cope for a long time and it is commonly at the time when the carer can no longer manage that the problem has to be shared. Often in the end it is the breakdown in the health of the carer that makes the condition known (see chapter 4).

The secret disease

An elderly dementing person living alone is only likely to be seen by a doctor when there is some sort of crisis. This may be when he starts wandering or when his neighbours notice things going wrong. In one study done in Edinburgh it was found that general practitioners were unaware of 80 per cent of the cases of moderately or severely demented old people on their lists. I have asked one very conscientious general practitioner about any patients with dementia in her practice. She knew of two. One was already dead but the surviving partner is still an active and articulate member of the Alzheimer's Disease Society; the other, one of her partner's patients, is still alive and a member of an influential and articulate local family. It is fair to assume that on this general practitioner's list there will be between thirty and forty dementing patients who have not been recognized and will not be noticed as long as the carer can cope. It is also interesting to note that the patients who are known both have an articulate near relative.

Loss of recent memory

Early in the disease there is loss of recent memory and it is this failure that accounts for many of the problems. The old man, or more commonly the old lady, will not remember the things that have occurred during the past week or day or even hours or minutes. It is this failure that makes any conversation so difficult because it may be impossible for the patient to remember what somebody else has just said. She may find it easier to dominate any conversation and talk about the things that she can remember such as her childhood, her parents and early friends. She will probably still remember these early experiences clearly and can therefore solve some of her present confusion by keeping the conversation firmly under her control. If somebody, such as a doctor or nurse, insists on taking over and asking what day of the week it is or what time of day, the old person can become very agitated and even angry because such questions begin to expose her confused mind.

Problems of a failing memory

A divorcee doing a full-time job, an only child and herself an old age pensioner, is anxious about her ninety-two-year-old mother. Her mother does still recognize her but fails to remember the things that have happened only an hour before. The old lady is still in her own home with an aged companion who is frail. The daughter goes to great lengths to have her mother to stay with her regularly so that the companion can have a much-needed rest.

She cooks all the things that her mother used to enjoy and takes her to the places that used to give her happiness; but the old lady now shows no appreciation of the trouble her daughter goes to, complains constantly, and when she gets back to her home again telephones her daughter to ask her when she is going to visit her and accuses her of neglect and doing nothing to please her. The daughter is naturally finding this a great strain and is tormented with doubts about what she should do. Her own health is suffering and she wonders whether she should go on doing all these things which apparently give her mother no pleasure and which she does not remember for even a few hours. Should she begin to consider her own health more and perhaps allow her mother to go into a home, knowing that she will feel guilty if this causes her mother distress and precipitates her death? There are no easy answers to these difficult and painful questions but it can help the carer to talk about them.

Problems in remembering the things which have happened recently may mean, for example, that a gas tap is turned on but not lit and this can, of course, be hazardous. As memory deteriorates skills such as reading, writing, telling the time, knowing how to use the telephone or write a cheque will go.

The general appearance of a person with dementia

Recently I was in a cathedral city in France and we walked past a group of French senior citizens being shown some of the sites by a guide. An old man with a shuffling walk, who was finding it difficult to keep up with the group, caught my attention. He knew he was part of the group and that he should be with them. It was a very hot day but he was wearing a large fur hat. He did have a walking stick but it was not helping his slow progress because he did not often put it on the ground but carried it like a small child would carry a rag doll. When he did manage to catch up with the group he stood on the edge and his expression was distant, lost and bewildered. He did not appear to understand what the guide was saying. Of course, I do not know that this old man had dementia but it seems probable. He showed many of the classic features of dementia including the *marche à petits pas* or little steps characteristic of this disease in its late stages (p. 42).

A common trait of the person who is developing dementia is the 'lost' look. There is always a sense of the unsureness of the child who has strayed into a strange adult world. The person whose inner sense of self is changing so drastically seems always to be looking around for some sort of reassurance and support and there may seem to be a fear of doing the wrong thing and a constant unspoken apology. There may sometimes be a look of bewilderment and at other times a lost and haunted look. Of course, everybody may show any of these emotions at different times, but in the demented they appear in inappropriate circumstances.

Intellectual deterioration

An eminent university professor who was about to retire and who planned to continue his research work in a laboratory specially provided for his retirement by the university started developing dementia. Although he could remember and talk about his earlier work and could help his biographer he was unable to concentrate on his present work or plan any of the research he was hoping to do. He has since deteriorated in many other ways but initially the intellectual changes were the most apparent.

A man or woman whose work depends on a good intellect and who has to make many decisions which may affect other people will show a deteriorating intellectual capacity early in the disease. The examples of this professor and of my husband who was a linguist and company chairman illustrated their respective early intellectual deterioration. Possibly this would not be so apparent early in a progressive dementia in a man who was doing manual labour.

Changes in personality *Behavioural*

Mrs R. changed from being a very dynamic person and the centre of a family with four adult children to living in a state of apathy with occasional outbursts of aggression. She was only fifty-two when these changes were first noted and although they were gradual they were progressive. At the onset she was an interested and interesting woman but became somebody totally lacking in energy, sitting listlessly in a chair looking at a wall. She just let life go on around her, she had no energy and her husband became bored. Her grown-up family attempted to help but nobody realized that her problem was dementia. Her husband withdrew from all social contacts because his wife could no longer cope and had become a social liability rather than an asset. The couple naturally became increasingly isolated and the husband had to cope with his own conflict of whether he should leave her and let her manage somehow. Finally he had a a breakdown, was no longer able to manage and care for her, and his wife had to be admitted to hospital. She lived only a few months longer and the family was left with a burden of guilt that they had not been able to cope.

Mrs C. is another example of a personality changing because of dementia. She is in her late fifties with a family of five grown-up children. She and her husband have been much involved in various sorts of charitable work and her altering behaviour causes much embarrassment. She often seems childlike as she rushes up to people and makes comments which are tactless and sometimes too honest. At other times she will go round saying 'I like you' to comparative strangers. She started looking untidy and was often inappropriately dressed. She would arrive late for important meetings and on occasion at social gatherings would drink too much. Her husband stopped her drinking any alcohol. She was quite accepting of his decision but the deterioration continued. Her husband finds it increasingly difficult to acknowledge that she is ill and not attempting to sabotage the structure of their social life.

Speech problems

Early in the disease words are forgotten and confused. Sometimes familiar words for very ordinary things, like shaving, may be used in unusual ways. My husband said that he must go to the other section (room) to cut the hair on his face (shave) (see p. 11). Late in the disease all intelligible speech may go and there will just be incoherent mumbling and disjointed words.

Movements

There is a general stiffness of muscles and difficulty in coordinating movements. Walking is stiff and can appear almost puppet-like. Characteristically the patient walks with small, stiff steps which are sometimes called *marche à petits pas*. All movements are difficult and those requiring more skill such as feeding become impossible. Familiar movements like putting on clothes become a lengthy ordeal partly because of muscle stiffness and muscle incoordination; but also forgetfulness about the next stage in the procedure being undertaken. Putting on a coat or tie becomes a long and complicated operation even with help.

An empty house

I recently heard a psychiatrist talking about the carer's problems after he had diagnosed dementia in her mother. All she could say was 'but where has she gone?' Relatives or close friends often have the feeling of the loss of somebody they love. The body is still there and occasionally a word or phrase which has the familiar sound of the person; but otherwise it can seem that the essential person has departed, leaving just a body and disabled mind behind.

Another daughter visited her dementing mother daily while she was still at home but eventually the old lady had to be admitted to a mental hospital and the daughter stopped visiting her. Perhaps she found the visits to the mental hospital too painful or she may have felt that an 'empty house' did not need her visits. Her mother had not recognized her for many months. The old lady died four months after admission to hospital and the daughter is now finding it difficult to forgive herself for not going to see her mother during the last months of her life.

4 / Recognition of the Patient

The shame of madness

We like to believe that we live in enlightened times and that there is no shame about having a mental illness. However, it is fair to assume that most people would prefer to have a physical illness and go into an ordinary hospital to have medical or surgical treatment than a mental illness and go into a mental hospital under the care of a psychiatrist. Age-old prejudice takes a long time to change. Many sorts of mental illness are now treatable but even these still have some stigma attached to them. Dementia is not treatable and therefore much of the deep-seated prejudice attaching to madness still lingers around it. If the old person's failing brain is made public, a relative may have many fantasies about what a psychiatrist will do, and removal to a mental hospital is one of the spectres that looms. In fact these are not the only ways of getting help and assistance sought in time can make it possible to look after the patient for longer at home. Fear about mental illness can be an additional reason that stops the carer asking for help.

Difficulties in recognition

Alzheimer's disease is not a disease in the usual medical model and as we have seen, its development tends to merge with the previous personality of the patient. Therefore its recognition as something abnormal which can be called a disease rather than

Carer

just oddness or eccentricity is a grey area. The recognition of Alzheimer's disease as a condition needing help depends more on the endurance of the nearest carer than the progress of the disease in the patient. The recognition of the condition is also inextricably tied up with the personality and resources of the carer and the amount of support received by the principal carer.

The conscientious carer is likely to suppress her own needs in order to satisfy the demands and requirements of the patient. The recognition of the patient's needs will sometimes only become apparent when the carer can no longer manage. This may be the reason why Alzheimer's disease often presents as a crisis.

The recognition of the patient and his assessment is important but the assessment and needs of the carer are of equal if not paramount importance. Alzheimer's disease is as yet an untreatable condition but the eventual recovery of the carer should not be jeopardized.

Presentation as crisis

Dementia of any sort, but particularly of the Alzheimer type, is frequently first recognized at a time of crisis. The disease will probably have been developing over several years and those in contact with it will have been tolerant of the changing personality and behaviour of the patient. A crisis will occur which will need the help of outside agencies. However, crisis management is not ideal because the reactions of professional advisers and the immediate help provided in such circumstances may not be of most benefit to the patient. More importantly, they may ignore the longer-term needs of the carer.

Why does dementia present as a crisis?
In some ways dementia is more like a child's reading problem than an ordinary physical or mental disease. The problem has

been around for a long time and does not in itself cause distress to the owner. It is only when there is conflict of some sort between the person with the problem and an outside measure of competence that it is recognized. For the child the problem can become apparent when changing to a different school or teacher. If the child could set up his own rules for literacy his problem would never become apparent. For the dementing patient it can be the onset of socially unacceptable behaviour or the removal of supportive neighbours and the moving in of less tolerant ones. John's dementia was containable as long as he had a supporting woman near, but not too near, who would tolerate his increasingly childish demands. I could be replaced by his cousin and he could keep control. The crisis came after he had his car accident and his cousin could no longer tolerate his demands. There was also the conflict between his dementing way of life and the law of the land. Neither the child with dyslexia nor the dementing patient will ever be the one who complains or asks for help. The stress will always be on the parent or the carer.

If dementia were a clearcut disease there could be recognized screening procedures, early diagnosis and planned management. Unfortunately, this is not the usual pattern and the majority of families keep the problem private until for one reason or another it is no longer possible to hide it. Many general practitioners do not know a lot about dementia and if approached may not be able to give information and guidance about practical management or legal or statutory help. There is no definitive assessment, diagnosis and treatment. It is understandable that the medical profession should have doubts about their ability to cope. Many doctors find it too threatening to deal with such a nebulous condition. There can be an unspoken and unwritten collusion that as long as the carers can cope it may be better to keep it secret. On the other hand, by doing so the carers may be driven by guilt or embarrassment to overstretch themselves physically or mentally and suffer a breakdown in their own health. In the long run this is the worst possible scenario for the quality of the remaining life of the patient.

Some of the common presenting crises

Guilt of the relatives or neighbours An old person who has been deteriorating over many years may be known to the neighbours and the tradesmen as needing care and support. The milkman is often one of the most practical and sensitive of social workers! The relatives, particularly if they live at a distance, can long remain in ignorance; and so can the professional carers. Yet there can be a sense of 'something ought to be done about this' and 'fancy relatives doing nothing to help this poor old man'. Suddenly one morning, the milk has not been taken off the doorstep, anxiety multiplies and it can become apparent that the responsibility is not entirely the milkman's or neighbour's and must now be shared. Occasionally, the apparent paranoia of the dementing person precipitates the crisis when the old person makes accusations of theft. Sometimes the bills are not being paid or the milkman cannot get his money and is told that the relatives have stolen it all. Again there can be a sudden decision that something must be done, and quickly.

Unacceptable behaviour I have one friend who coped quite nobly with a dementing mother in her own small flat and under incredibly trying and demanding conditions. She managed until the old lady became critically confused during the night and repeatedly mistook the laundry basket for the toilet. Suddenly the whole thing was no longer bearable and her mother was sent to a psychogeriatric hospital. An earlier request for help could have made a different management possible and maybe my friend was too caring and too conscientious.

Another old lady was managing adequately in an ordinary old people's home until she decided to go for walks outside during the night with nothing on. The home could cope with the wandering but not with the nakedness. In both these instances the crisis was not caused by a sudden deterioration in the patient's illness but in the way a social limit for the carers had been overstepped.

An accident My elderly mother, whose mind had been failing over many years, managed adequately in an upstairs flat on her own until she had an accident. She had had raised blood pressure for many years and during the past few years had suffered a number of TIAs (see p. 34). During one TIA she fell, fractured her hip and was admitted to hospital. The time she spent in a busy hospital ward and loss of control over her own life precipitated an acute confusional state and services had then to be organized.

I was one of the main carers in this instance and had already had the experience of caring for my husband while he had dementia. I realized the importance of leaving as much control as possible in the hands of the patient, and with my sister was able to set up an intricate home support system so that my mother was able to return home and survive in her own flat.

Ignorance of professional helpers If the general practitioner is ignorant about dementia and prefers not to get involved, it is likely that a crisis will occur eventually. At that moment the doctor will try to get the patient off his hands as fast as possible. He can get the help of an expert, for example a psychiatrist. They may then make a home visit and sort it all out. Some general practitioners will go to great lengths to help carers and facilitate support but others do not know what local help might be available and how to mobilize it. Some older doctors, who have not had experience of managing dementia, can find that mental illness is frightening and threatening and prefer not to get involved.

A preventive crisis Sometimes a previously uncommunicative but supporting family is going away on holiday, is nervous about what will happen if the old man is found wandering around at night, and is prompted to demand help from somebody at very short notice. This type of crisis, although understandable, is unlikely to produce the best long-term solution for the patient.

The variations of this sort of crisis are infinite but basically the circumstances of the nearest carers are about to change and they are prompted to ask for help – often at short notice.

Can crises be prevented? In essence, all these crises have more to do with the exhaustion or exasperation of the carer than a sudden down-turn in the state of the patient. The prevention of crises and the provision of help and support for the carer at a much earlier stage depends on the willingness of the carer to discuss her difficulties with somebody. The 'somebody' clearly needs to be a person with a good understanding of the problem, who realizes that the carer's needs are of more immediate importance that those of the patient. The general practitioner could be such a person but he will need to make some time available to unravel the problem. No quick diagnosis and treatment will be possible.

The health visitor or practice nurse could be the right person. Their time may be more flexible, even though they may be busy people. They will, however, need knowledge and understanding to provide the sort of help and support that are necessary.

Most importantly, the carer needs to be honest about her own needs and begin to set some sort of agenda of what must be done to help her. If she is tired physically, mentally and emotionally and full of feelings of guilt and inadequacy, she is going to find it extremely difficult to be clear-minded and prepared to think about her own needs. It is therefore important to look for help *before* you are at the end of your tether, when you are still in a position to make reasonably rational judgements.

5 / Assessment of the Patient

Dementias of the Alzheimer type do not look like most other diseases because they tend to develop very slowly. At times Alzheimer sufferers may look a bit like a caricature of the original person and therefore the time when a 'diagnosis' is required may never arrive. However, as and when the carer can cope no longer, or the patient is brought to the doctor's attention through outside pressure, an attempt must be made to assess, diagnose and then manage the patient. Usually the most important part of the whole process will be assessing the needs of the carer and finding and mobilizing suitable and adequate support. Obviously the patient's needs are of great importance but these are more apparent than those of the carer.

How is an assessment made?

The person with dementia usually has no idea that he is diseased in any way and may avoid what was for him normal contact with the medical profession. Perhaps in John's case, his refusal to see his general practitioner was a sort of acknowledgement that there was something wrong with him. When he was 'well' he consulted doctors frequently but when he was dementing he used his annual private medical check-up as evidence that there was absolutely nothing wrong with his health. He was only assessed as a patient for whom something needed to be done when his cousin, who was near, and myself, who was distant, could no longer carry the burden. I had already had a breakdown and I believe at the time of John's assessment his cousin was near to one.

Mrs A. is surrounded by a very supportive family and has been deteriorating over a number of years. She is a gentle person and her assessment has been done by guile because the family is in the special position of having friends who are medical practitioners. The diagnosis has been made and somebody has been employed to look after her at home but no sort of coercion has been necessary.

Role of the general practitioner

A general practitioner who knows his patients and who works in a team with a practice nurse and a health visitor is possibly best placed to make an early diagnosis of a dementing person and then to offer appropriate help and support to the carers. Confirmation of the diagnosis and exclusion of other treatable causes of dementia may need specialist help, which can then be sought at the appropriate time. If general practitioners felt more confident about being in such a key position they could be of inestimable value to all those concerned in the management of a dementing person.

The general practitioner can, if he or the family feels it to be necessary, arrange a home visit by a psychiatrist, geriatrician or psychogeriatrician. The exact title of the consultant called in is not as important as his or her known interest in all the problems associated with dementia. The 'expert' clinical diagnosis of dementia is seldom as important as the wisdom of the professional helper in arranging the right support for the family and helping them to adjust to a tragic situation. The availability of doctors with special experience and knowledge varies from one part of the country to another. A psychiatric nurse or social worker may be asked to make a preliminary or subsequent assessment. The diagnosis is as important for the carer as for the patient, if not more so, because it enables her to relinquish some of the responsibility on to other shoulders and makes it more respectable to accept help.

The assessment of the patient is best done at home where the consultant, accompanied by the general practitioner, can see what the patient is like in his own 'patch', interview friends, relatives or other carers, and have the opportunity of seeing the whole problem at the grass roots level. Further tests may be necessary and sometimes it is desirable for the patient to have further assessment or diagnostic tests at hospital. From the patient's point of view these are better done as an outpatient than as an inpatient.

I shall not attempt in the space of this small book to give details about all the possible ways of assessing the patient and attempting to measure the degree of the problem. What follows is a brief outline. Details of where further information can be found are given in the appendix.

What investigations should be done?

There is continuing medical debate about how extensively a patient with dementia should be investigated; but there is complete agreement that some investigations are obligatory to establish whether there is any possibility of a treatable cause of the dementia. To allow anybody to dement when they could have been effectively treated would indeed be a tragedy. It must be stressed that such conditions are rare and the chances of them being missed are small. Note must be made of alcohol use and abuse in the past as well as the present. Alcohol abuse can cause a Korsakoff psychosis with irreversible loss of short-term memory or alcohol dementia which can be partially reversible if the alcohol is stopped.

Essential investigations include:

1. Taking a full history of what has happened to the patient, possibly over a period of several years. This can take a lot of time because the patient himself must be asked and will probably only be able to give a limited and distorted version of the events that have led up to the present assessment. An account must also be obtained from the nearest carer and possibly other relatives and friends and neighbours who have been involved. This 'history taking' is an essential part of any assessment, is best done in the patient's own home and should ideally be done without any pressure of time.

A history of a past depressive illness should be noted because it may give a clue to the patient's present condition. Depressive illness is common in older people but it can usually be distinguished from early dementia by the recognition of previous depressive episodes. The characteristics of depressive illness are early morning waking, improvement in mood by evening, loss of appetite and weight and the general feeling of hopelessness. The mental confusion that can occur during a depressive illness in an older person is usually much more variable than in a progressive dementia of the Alzheimer type, and has been called 'pseudo-dementia'. It may only be possible to diagnose such a condition in retrospect when there is complete recovery after psychiatric treatment for the underlying depressive illness.

2. General observations of the patient's behaviour may show that he is restless, confused and out of touch with his surroundings. If he is paranoid he may show agitation and some anger that there are strange people in his home. He may feel threatened by the situation.

3. A general physical examination of the patient is done to exclude physical diseases including anaemia. The blood pressure

will be measured and there will be some assessment of sight and hearing. A full examination of the nervous system will be made looking particularly for localized neurological signs. Observations will be made of the patient's walking. In advancing dementia the patient may shuffle along with very short steps. He can be so stiff that he seems to find both walking and sitting difficult. The physical examination can also show the evidence of incontinence either of urine or faeces or both.

If the assessment is done late in the course of the disease, as it was for John, speech may be confused with no memory of the names of people or objects. There may be only jibberish or indecipherable mumbling.

4. Some general examination of the patient's mental state will always be done. There are now many schemes for getting a reasonably objective measurement and one of the currently favoured ones is the Cambridge Mental Disorders of the Elderly Examination (CAMDEX). This incorporates measurements of both physical and a wide variety of mental functions to give an overall measurement of the patient's current state.

5. Laboratory investigations must be done to exclude the rare but treatable causes of dementia including any deficiency in the working of the thyroid gland and a low level of vitamin B_{12} in the blood. The blood examination will include checks for anaemia and a general electrolyte survey. Tests for syphilis and the function of the liver may be included.

6. Radiological investigations will usually include X-rays of the skull and chest. A CT scan of the head is seldom helpful unless there is the possibility of a brain tumour. It is indeed usually possible to demonstrate that the brain is shrinking but this knowledge is not of any practical use to the patient or his carers. Magnetic resonance imaging (MRI) can also be used to

demonstrate the brain changes typical of Alzheimer's disease; but unless the patient becomes part of a research project or there is doubt about the diagnosis, there is little benefit to the patient or carers in carrying out these investigations. In addition the patient is likely to become more disturbed by anything which upsets his 'normal' routine. Unless there is good reason for doing a lumbar puncture, it should be avoided because it can be particularly upsetting for the patient.

Follow-up to the assessment

Following the assessment of the patient there should be an opportunity for the carer to meet with the general practitioner and possibly the consultant to discuss the next steps. It is unlikely that the investigations will have shown anything apart from the confirmation of Alzheimer's disease. In the unlikely event of a treatable type of dementia being found, treatment will, of course, be provided. It may be possible that the patient with Alzheimer's disease can stay at home if sufficient support is provided.

Alternatively day care or short or longer-term residential care may seem more appropriate. Drugs can help some of the symptoms including restlessness. Management of the patient is discussed in chapter 6.

6 / Management of the Patient

Crisis management or planned management?

For the reasons outlined in chapter 4, Alzheimer's disease is most likely to be recognized and some sort of management started at a time of crisis. It would be preferable for both the patient and the principal carer if management could be started at a chosen time, but there are many difficulties. The first is the problem of recognizing the point at which a rather confused or difficult person, who has to be tolerated, becomes a patient with Alzheimer's disease who needs management. The second is the failure of the carer to recognize her own need for help. She may allow herself to be driven to the point of a breakdown in her own physical, mental or emotional health. At that point she appears to be the patient and the real sufferer remains unrecognized. This is probably a common occurrence: I know of people to whom it has happened, and it happened to me.

I believe the main reason for the carer's failure to recognize her own need is that she is already going through the process of bereavement. The loss of the partner has already begun. The companionship is going, the quality of the relationship is deteriorating and he is changing from an adult to a dependent child. There is already, for the carer, a sense of incompleteness and loss although the patient's body is still present. The self-image of the partner changes as the patient disintegrates. The process of bereavement has started and it progresses relentlessly as the patient's condition worsens; but it is not possible for the carer to begin to grieve, and it is difficult to admit to or share any of this distress. All the reactions of bereavement including the numbness, disbelief, feelings of isolation, confusion and anger can be present but are apparently inexplicable because the patient is there.

At this time, the carer is being called upon to identify the patient's problem. This can seem like a further demand that is impossible to meet. However, it is important not only for the present welfare of the patient but for the longer-term physical, mental and emotional health of the carer that she should be helped and encouraged to meet this demand.

Setting the agenda

It is all too easy for the carer through her confused feelings, including inadequacy and guilt and a state of chronic exhaustion, to remain unaware of the key role she must play in the life of the patient. She must try to understand her importance and find the courage to 'set the agenda' for the management of the patient. It will help clarify her thoughts to talk over all the problems with other relatives, friends, and a sympathetic general practitioner or health visitor. She is the one best placed to decide how much she can cope with and what help she needs. She must try not to feel frightened, diffident or ashamed about putting her own needs at the top of the agenda. The whole plan will need frequent revision if it is to remain realistic in coping with the patient's progressive deterioration.

The carer needs to ask herself some specific questions. It may help to write these down with the answers and if she is in doubt about relevant questions and honest answers, to discuss them with a near relative or trusted friend. Questions should include: Am I well enough physically and mentally to go on coping? Can I go on coping with the patient living in the house with me? If he goes on living at home what help do I need now? Are there any special problems with which I should like help? Would it make a difference if he was away from me for one or more days a week? Would it help if I could be sure of two hours a day away from him? I can only make suggestions about relevant questions but these are an indication of those to which answers should be found.

Next on the agenda will be the needs of the patient. What is best for the patient? Try asking the patient. It can all too easily be assumed that because a person is dementing he no longer has any idea of what he wants. Try asking him where he wants to live and he will usually say that he wants to stay at home. It is great to have such a straightforward answer in the middle of confusion but now one has to balance this against the well-being of the carer. How much can she stand and in all honesty what help does she require in order to survive? The majority of dementing people do want to stay in their own home and in one survey it was shown that at least 60 per cent manage to do so.

Admission to hospital is contemplated by the majority of families only as a last resort; but in one survey it was found that only a quarter of those looking after mildly demented relatives and a fifth of those looking after more severely demented relatives had, in fact, discussed their problems with the general practitioner. The carers did not ask for help because they thought that there was no possibility of being helped.

An acceptable level of risk

Once a person starts dementing there will be an increased risk of some sort of accident, particularly if he lives alone or spends any time alone. Some of the risks can and should be eliminated but it is not possible to remove all of them without confining the dementing person to bed, which in any case would increase the risk of bronchopneumonia. The hazards to be eliminated include rugs on slippery surfaces, trailing flexes, unsafe electrical equipment, access to garden and household poisons and an unlocked medicine cupboard. Gas appliances will always have some risk but modern automatic lighting gas stoves are safer than those that have to be lit with a match.

I had thought a lot about carers and caring because of my experience with John before my elderly mother broke her hip, was taken into hospital and became mentally confused. She had been developing multi-infarct dementia following a number of TIAs. In an objective way, she was unable to survive on her own in a first-floor flat with no lift and no sort of supervision. She could only walk with the help of a frame and could not navigate the stairs to her front door. However, in the middle of her confusion there was only one thing that she was sure that she wanted and that was to get back to her own home. With much research, organization and choice of easily operated electronic magic this was made possible. At one point a home care organizer asked me if I was confident that my mother would be safe during all the hours she would be on her own. The answer was obviously 'no', but we took the risk. I was not asked to sign a document to say that I would accept the risk on her behalf! All life is risky and it does not become less so for the dementing patient. At the time of writing this book my mother is still managing on her own although precariously.

Part of the carer's role is being able to balance and accept such risks. Neither must the carer feel too guilty when something goes wrong as inevitably it will.

Qualities of the carer

Common sense is the most valuable attribute of the carer and she must understand that dementia is not a disease that should be diagnosed, treated and cured by experts. That is not possible. The carer needs to feel confident that the common-sense approach is the right one. At the same time it must also be understood that the condition of dementia is not normal ageing but some type of distorted and accelerated change in brain tissue. Dementia is not something that is going to happen to all of us as we get older, and there is no need to be fearful that it will, but living close to another's disintegration can feel very threatening to one's own integrity.

Fatigue, anger and exasperation are as normal in caring for an old person with dementia as in caring for a small child who is being extremely difficult. It is better to admit and even express anger than to keep it bottled up. Ordinary care and patience and kindness – even a touch of honest anger – are what the patient most needs. The nearest and most familiar person to the patient is the one ideally placed to supply the care, but this should never be at the risk of destroying the carer's own health.

The common-sense approach includes making sure that the patient has spectacles to see as well as possible, but at the same time understanding that 'reading' may not be possible because although the eyes can see the written words, the brain can no longer understand them. Hearing should be approached in the same way. A simple hearing aid and batteries are important but getting a very sophisticated device in the hope of making the patient better able to understand speech and the meaning of other sounds, and be more like his old self, will lead to inevitable disappointment. Another practical help for daily living are well-fitting dentures which are important for chewing food and for speaking.

It is more important to listen, or at least appear to listen, than to keep talking to the patient. Communication and instruction should be kept to a minimum and should never be confusing. One clock that shows the correct time is a lot more use than John's fifteen clocks which all showed different times. Simple written instructions in large print, and perhaps with simple illustrations or diagrams, about turning on and off lights or the way to the toilet can be very helpful; but again they must be kept to a minimum and be about essential functions. John enjoyed electronic wizardry and kept instructions for himself on mini-cassettes; but in the end things got so complicated with tapes explaining where the other tapes were that it added to his increasing confusion. The carer needs to be able to edit out some of the complications and keep all the instructions relevant to the patient's current lifestyle.

Arguing with the patient is an exhausting, frustrating and useless occupation. There are moments when it is better to assume that you and the patient are speaking different languages without an interpreter present. With this sort of understanding it can be easier to accept the different ways in which you and the patient are viewing the world and each other without the need for useless entanglement and further distress. You know that your languages are mutually incomprehensible even if he does not!

Psychological reality-orientation is the technical way of saying what I am trying to describe. It is what the normally competent parent does instinctively for a child and the carer needs to do for the dementing patient – even without knowing the technical term. It means helping the patient to get on with his ordinary life in the most real and practicable way feasible and with the minimum of fuss. He can then live in as socially acceptable a way as possible with all his faculties failing. You must accept the reality that this is indeed second childhood for the patient but the direction is growing down and not growing up.

Choosing the help

Having assessed her own and the patient's needs with help from friends and professionals, the carer next needs to be informed about and choose, with adequate guidance, those sources of help which will be of most use to her and the patient. These sources are described in the next chapter.

7 / Sources of Help

In a bureaucratic society and an increasingly bureaucratic health service, needs must be identified and labelled before help is available. You have begun to identify your needs as those of the carer of a patient with Alzheimer's disease by making a list of relevant questions and possible answers to them (see p. 58). You will now be in a better position to start the search for the help that will be most suitable for you and for the patient with Alzheimer's disease. The availability of suitable help will vary from one area to another and you may need to use some imagination and persistence to find what is best for you. You are most likely to start your search by consulting your general practitioner because he is easily identifiable.

The role of the general practitioner

In the United Kingdom everybody has or is entitled to have a general practitioner. He can and should be the key person in recognizing the condition of the patient with Alzheimer's disease and ideally, the chief coordinator in the provision of practical and emotional support for the carer and the patient. However, in order to fulfil these roles the general practitioner needs to be fully conversant with the state of the patient and the carer. The carer is the only possible provider of the necessary information and she must be honest about the real state of the patient and about her own needs; and the general practitioner must listen with an open mind and realize that he can do a great deal to provide information and coordinate the available support services. He can start by introducing the health visitor, who is probably attached to his practice, to the carer. He will already have played a major part in the assessment and diagnosis of the patient and will possibly have made a referral to a consultant.

Unfortunately a patient, in this case probably the carer, finds it easier to talk about one particular physical problem, and it is easier for many general practitioners to give a solution to such a problem. It is much more difficult for both of them to sit down in a relaxed way and discuss a patient who is dementing and the possible long-term strategies for the best-quality survival of the carer and the patient. Therefore, there can be an unhelpful collusion between the carer and the general practitioner. The carer does not want to be honest about the changes in the patient, particularly if it is her spouse, and the general practitioner is often unhappy and feels inadequate in managing a patient with dementia. With such barriers and within the limited time of a normal appointment, it is easier for the carer to talk about one physical problem. For example, the carer says that the patient does not seem able to see properly and the general practitioner arranges for an expert opinion on the state of his eyes. Both have avoided the problem that the deteriorating mental state of the patient makes understanding of the written word impossible. Many other symptoms may be presented in such a way including hearing, digestive problems or cardiovascular disease.

If the general practitioner is made aware of the changing mental state of the patient many such unnecessary and unhelpful hospital attendances could be avoided. Such referrals are not only time-wasting but can be positively harmful. Any hospital attendance and particularly an admission, an anaesthetic and numerous drugs can precipitate further confusion and accelerate the process of disintegration. Sometimes a hospital admission or operation will be unavoidable but should only be undertaken after serious and honest discussion between the general practitioner or consultant and the relatives. A balanced view must be reached and many surgical procedures, far from relieving the problems that already exist, will only make the overall condition of the patient worse. It is the general practitioner, in his role as overall guide, who can best advise the carer.

The health visitor

There will probably be a health visitor attached to your general practitioner's practice. She is a trained nurse who has a specialist qualification in health visiting and whose experience is geared to preventive care. You cannot expect her to come up with some magic solution but she may have more time to listen and be able to discuss with you the most important problems at that moment. She will be a good source of information, counsel and support. She will also be able to put you in touch with all the other statutory services including social workers, occupational therapists, Meals on Wheels, the incontinence laundry service and the district nurses. She will give you information about the local voluntary services including the Alzheimer's Disease Society, Age Concern and Help the Aged. She will know about the local availability of day centres and residential care. If a dementing person is living on his own, the more regular help he has the better it will be for him. Visitors arriving with a clear reason and for an obvious benefit will help him keep in touch with the day of the week and the time of day as well as providing him with necessary care, food, service and companionship. Neighbours are likely to remain more supportive if the whole burden of care is not falling on them.

Nurses and nursing care

Your general practitioner will be able to arrange nursing care if it is necessary, which will probably be unlikely until late in the disease. Bathing or giving an enema may be the occasions for nursing help.

Home care assistants

The home care organizer will come to the house and assess the need for help. Previously, such help was called 'home help' and included housework; but at the time of writing this book the home care assistant will give many services though excluding routine housework. She will get the patient dressed in the morning, leave food ready, and care for him in many ways including shopping and collecting the pension. She may return later to undress him and put him to bed. She is allowed to wash but not bath him and she is not allowed to do any chiropody including care of toenails. District nurses will call and a chiropodist will do a home visit if the patient is not able to get out. Such help can be an invaluable support; but there is a shortage of people to do this work in many areas and therefore time may have to be severely restricted. Payment is according to means.

Occupational therapist

She can do an assessment of the patient's house and make suggestions about suitable aids and alterations. A ramp to the front door if the patient is in a wheelchair or stair rails can be of great help. She will do an assessment of the bathroom and arrange aids such as a special toilet seat, rails or a hoist for the bath. She will have a fund of experience and sources of information about all the gadgetry which can make day-to-day living easier for both the carer and the patient. The carer needs first to do her personal assessment of all the things that are difficult and then ask if there is any possibility of help.

Meals on Wheels

This service is available throughout the UK and is normally provided five days a week. In some areas, a seven-day service is available if necessary. Although an old person may complain about the food provided it is usually of excellent quality and value. Apart from providing food the service can also provide contact and brief companionship as well as a dependable cause for complaint!

Domiciliary hairdressing

Many hairdressers will do home visits on a regular basis for men or women, and in my experience a competent hairdresser can also be an expert therapist in the management of the dementing person. It is worth setting up a regular visit because it means that the patient will look better and there will be another regular and employed visitor who is performing a useful function.

Day centres

Some day centres are organized for the daily care of the patient and can be of immense help to the hard-pushed carer, although, as with a small child starting at nursery school, the initial time spent away from the best-known carer can be very traumatic. Parting can be emotionally difficult and there can be many delaying tactics before the farewell in the morning. However, once there are familiar faces at the centre it can become a happy and acceptable arrangement. The arrangement can be for one or more days a week and is as useful for the relief of the carer as for the occupation of the patient.

Some day centres are essentially short-term treatment centres with a full range of services including physiotherapy, chiropody and occupational therapy.

Residential care

The time may come when the carer needs a temporary or permanent break from the non-stop demands of the dementing person and the wearying and unceasing responsibility. Your general practitioner, the health visitor, local social services department or the Alzheimer's Disease Society will help you. They can advise you on the best place for temporary admission to a hospital or nursing home or guide you in finding a more permanent place for the patient to stay.

Use of drugs

Although much research is being done on drugs that may slow down or relieve mental deterioration in Alzheimer's disease there are still no drugs that treat the condition. The monthly newsletter from the Alzheimer's Disease Society gives excellent updates on the state of present knowledge and an accurate digest of the reliable and reported medical research.

Drugs can be used to control symptoms including constipation, sleeplessness, aggressive behaviour and severe agitation. You must observe the changing condition of the patient and discuss it with your doctor. He will then guide you on suitable drugs which might help but you will have to be realistic and honest about the most troublesome problems and realize that they are unlikely to be completely solvable.

Useful gadgets

An identity disc worn on the wrist is a valuable piece of equipment for the patient who tends to wander. Just the name and the telephone number should be engraved on the disc. Sometimes it may be necessary to fit door locks that the patient is unable to open, but this move may cause the patient much distress and should be considered carefully.

If the patient is still able to be left alone for periods and can understand its use, an AIDCALL alarm worn as a pendant round the neck can be advisable.

The Alzheimer's Disease Society

Any carer should join the society and possibly one of its local support groups. There are those who will welcome the activities of such a group and those who prefer to remain more isolated. The society produces an excellent, well-researched, accurate and informative monthly newsletter and a range of regularly updated leaflets. The society is in a much better position to provide information about available benefits and resources than a book such as this because facts change so fast. It can be surprisingly difficult to find all the available sources of help even if you consider yourself a normally enterprising and well-organized person, and contact with the Alzheimer's Disease Society can be a most fruitful source of information. You must then be prepared to follow up every lead and if necessary be very persistent and demanding. You know what help you need, such help may well be available in your locality and you are probably entitled to a great deal of it under the National Health Service or social services.

Other voluntary organizations

You can either contact such voluntary organizations as Age

Concern and Help the Aged to discover what help they may be able to give you; or you can first consider your needs and then use the voluntary organizations as possible suppliers of those needs. The Samaritans can be of help in an emergency and you may have other local counselling organizations. Addresses of such organizations are given in the appendix.

Sources of mental and emotional help

Being the carer for a patient with Alzheimer's disease provides an opportunity for understanding more about being a carer. It can also be a time for understanding more about being cared for. During bereavement, and Alzheimer's disease is a continuing bereavement, there is a need to accept help and care. This time of caring can, therefore, be a time of learning and greater self-understanding for the carer.

It is easy for good carers to know the patient's needs so well that it hastens their progress to childlike dependency. Most of us can become rebellious when taken over in such a way. I have been angry when a powerful carer has assumed to know my needs better than I did; but this is what I was doing myself when I sorted out John's needs, and what I could easily have done when my mother became confused. Certainly I had to take over responsibility for John, and this is a normal pattern when somebody is disintegrating. However, the carer can be gratifying her own needs as well as those of the patient; and I had to look at my own arrogance in assuming I knew what was best for somebody else.

Who can help the carer?

If you are a practising member of any faith, your minister, priest or other religious leader may well be a source of help and guidance. I happen to be a Christian and to have been reared in the Anglican tradition. I have had the most constructive help from several priests. You have to be registered with one general practitioner and then only go to that one for help. In one sense, if you are a member of the Church of England, your local vicar is your spiritual general practitioner. However, there is nothing unethical about going for confidential help or advice to another priest. You may hear of a particularly helpful one from a friend or go to a retreat and meet one.

Your minister will be able to see the dementing patient and help the carer, by offering her the chance to share all her pent-up emotions. It is normal for a carer to feel anger. It is not wrong to feel angry and it is much less destructive to be able to admit the anger than to feel it must be disguised at all costs.

The minister of a given religion will be able to offer the particular help of that faith. For the Christian it will be penance and absolution, laying on of hands and the Eucharist. There will also be an opportunity to think and talk about the meaning of dying and death and the ceremonies that go with them. Priests know a lot more about death and dying than doctors.

If a carer can talk honestly and openly to a spiritual adviser, she may come to understand more about how caring satisfies her own needs. Some carers do need to go on coping. A strong man caring for his wife with dementia may discover within himself hidden gifts of tenderness which he can now use to good effect. Perhaps for the first occasion in his life he can not only cry but cry in public, and those watching will think of him as a courageous man and not somebody to be despised. He has discovered a hidden and almost lost talent, and in a strange way caring for his wife will give him a greater richness in his own life.

The Good Samaritan

The Bible can be a source of help and I am sure that other

religious writing with which I am not familiar can be of equal support. The parable of the Good Samaritan seems to me a good role model for the carer. It will probably be familiar to most readers but I will quote here the version from St Luke's Gospel in the Jerusalem Bible.

> (A lawyer asked) 'And who is my neighbour?' Jesus replied, 'A man was once on his way down from Jerusalem to Jericho and fell into the hands of brigands; they took all he had, beat him and then made off, leaving him half dead. Now a priest happened to be travelling down the same road, but when he saw the man he passed by on the other side. In the same way a Levite who came to the place saw him, and passed by on the other side. But a Samaritan traveller who came upon him was moved with compassion when he saw him. He went up and bandaged his wounds, pouring oil and wine on them. He then lifted him on to his own mount, carried him to the inn and looked after him. Next day, he took out two denarii and handed them to the innkeeper. "Look after him," he said, "and on my way back I will make good any expense you have." '

Perhaps this is the ideal model for the carer. He assessed the injured man's needs and was then a good steward of his own resources of time, talents and money. He did not hang around and make any attempt at becoming indispensable. He did all he could and then went off and got on with his own life. He certainly had no great desire to be needed. He was not blind to his own needs and therefore blind to those of the wounded person. And he would not have become a burnt-out carer!

Carers all run the risk of overextending themselves and ending up as emptied of personhood as the dementing person they are caring for. Observing another's needs and ignoring one's own is commendable in the short term but leads to intolerable and self-destructive stress in the longer term.

Self-help groups

A self-help group can be a source of personal help for the carer; but of course the word 'carer' covers a multitude of unique individuals. No two carers will be alike and that must never be forgotten. We can only cope and care to the limits of our own abilities and we should not seek to emulate anybody else. So much in our contemporary world is competitive and therefore comparative. This can become very destructive and threatening for the individual. 'If she can cope with all that work and worry, why can't I?' can so quickly be translated into 'If I can't cope with that much and she can, then I am not of much use.' If a self-help group is available and you find it good, that is fine. But a carer must not allow herself to become part of some moral auction.

Help with the legal implications of dementia

A dementing person becomes forgetful and disorganized. He may not have made a will and probably will not know how much money he has or where it is. John had a habit of keeping small amounts of money in many different countries of the world and it is very unlikely that I shall ever find these secret caches. By the time he died he was totally out of touch with such things. The ability to manage day-to-day and more long-term financial affairs will not all go at once but will disintegrate slowly. The progressive deterioration in the ability to cope should be anticipated and plans made accordingly. This is not a morbid activity but an essential one for the well-being of the patient and possibly of the spouse. A small amount of clear thinking, some good professional advice and determined action can save a lot of painful situations when the dementing person is totally unable to manage the chaos. It can also make the management of his affairs after his death a lot less painful.

Has the dementing person made a will?

Even if you are the spouse you may not know if the dementing patient has made a will or if so where it is kept. This is particularly likely if the patient always tended to be secretive about money matters. The patient must, in the eyes of the law, be of 'testamentary capacity' in order to make a valid will. If he does not realize that he is making a will, and is not aware of the amount and nature of the property at his disposal and his relationship with those to whom he is being expected to leave it, he is no longer in a fit mental state to be making a will.

If possible the will should be made while the patient is still of 'testamentary capacity' but if this is not possible, a solicitor will be able to advise you. If during the course of his dementia the patient has made a will which is not believed to have been in accordance with his judgement before he deteriorated, it is possible to have it changed after his death with the agreement of the main beneficiaries of the will, by a Deed of Variation.

There are many problems here. Alzheimer's disease is of such insidious onset that it can be extremely difficult to decide when the patient was last of testamentary capacity. Trying to rewrite a will after the death of a demented patient, when all those nearest are in the early stages of bereavement, is an emotional minefield. This process should be avoided if at all possible. If the patient's affairs have been taken over by the Court of Protection it can be asked that the will should be found and deposited with the Court. The Receiver can then have access to it and the problem of rewriting it referred to the Court. If the patient has not made a will, the Court of Protection can be asked to do it before the patient's death.

Court of Protection

If there is no power of attorney and the patient is not able to manage his affairs, application must be made to the Court of Protection who can manage the patient's affairs on a short term or lifetime commitment. It is an efficient and compassionate organization. A relative or friend can become Receiver for the patient under the Court of Protection; or failing this a solicitor may be appointed. I was Receiver for John and had a named contact at the office of the Court of Protection; so that when circumstances changed there was no delay in getting advice and help and the release of money for John's benefit. An application can either be made direct to the Personal Application Branch of the Court or through a solicitor of your choosing.

Power of attorney

A person who is dementing but still able to manage his own affairs can sign a 'power of attorney' giving broad authority or limited powers to somebody of the patient's choosing to look after his affairs. This does not need to become fully operational until the mental state of the patient warrants it. This is a very valuable procedure because it means that the patient has the right to choose the person who will handle his affairs when necessary; and that there need be no delay in having access to the patient's financial resources when it should be necessary to sell a house or pay private nursing home fees.

8 / Terminal Illness and Death

I have heard Alzheimer's disease described as a 'slow good-bye' or as an 'ongoing bereavement'. These seem accurate descriptions of the long-lasting pain of watching somebody you once knew as a rather different person, change and disintegrate. You watch and wait and are unable to help. It is inappropriate to grieve or mourn while the body is still there but the essential spirit of the person seems to have disappeared. One woman said, 'She is not really my mum because the mum I knew has died.' I heard somebody else say, 'I married for better and for worse but this is not the person I married so am I still tied by my marriage vows?' These are devastating problems and they go on for a long time. The length of this ongoing bereavement is an essential factor in the period of time that the carer will need to recover after the death of the patient.

What do patients with Alzheimer's disease die from?

The disease can go on for so many years that the question of death of the body as well as the death that has already occurred of the mind and spirit always seems a long way distant. In fact life expectancy is always reduced and the end when it does come can be surprisingly rapid. Loss of weight nearly always does occur late in the course of the disease and in the last months of life wasting away of the body can be rapid and profound. A patient is more likely to fall because he is weak and unsteady; and because he will be progressively less active and sometimes forced to remain seated in a chair or lying in a bed, he is more likely to get a chest infection followed by bronchopneumonia. Bronchopneumonia is a very merciful and peaceful end, but it may be necessary to say to the doctor in charge that you do not want antibiotics to be given. I did do that and John's death from bronchopneumonia was unbelievably peaceful and serene. Ultimately the doctor's decisions will be made in the best interests of the patient; and in this instance a doctor will usually listen to a near relative.

Where will death occur?

Most people if they could state a preference would, I believe, prefer to die in their own home and bed. There is no reason for somebody dying from dementia to be an exception. Death is a normal process and one best accomplished within the family. Of course, if the patient is already in residential care he will normally stay there; but if you have managed to keep him at home, that will usually be the best place for him to die. The process of dying is less familiar to most individuals and families now than it was 100 years ago. Fewer children die and so most of us have not experienced death at close quarters until our parents die; and more deaths at an earlier age take place in a hospital or hospice with experts in charge. It is therefore easy to assume that dying needs some sort of special professional care. As a doctor I had seen many people who were going to die, and many dead bodies, but I had never shared anybody's death until I shared John's. Sharing his death made me feel that it is good and right that the nearest relative should be there during dying. It must be a lonely process and one during which the dying person is clearly very vulnerable. He needs the companionship of the person who has been, perhaps a very long time ago in Alzheimer's disease, closest to him in a loving relationship.

If special help, such as pain relief, is necessary, a doctor can be called. A district nurse will be available for any nursing help such as bathing, turning or changing the bed. You can be the person who is there to comfort, give sips of drink or moisten the mouth when necessary. You should, if possible, have somebody else in the house so that you can be looked after and fed. You will need rest and sleep and somebody to relieve you at such times. Another relative or friend is probably the best person to help you; but otherwise your doctor, nurse or religious adviser will be able to make suggestions for your support.

Death is not optional

If the patient is a practising religious person you may well have been in touch with his priest or other religious leader. This will have given you an opportunity to talk about death and dying. You may have been able to ask him or your doctor about a good and reliable funeral director. It is not morbid to think and talk about this in advance; and you will probably feel a lot less apprehensive about the inevitable death that will occur once you have thought about the practical arrangements. As soon as the death does occur you contact your doctor and then the funeral director who will guide you through all the formalities. A good funeral director can be a competent guide and compassionate counsellor at such a time.

If the body is laid out at home by a nurse, it can be beneficial for the family and close friends to see it there. The person can look very peaceful, much younger and more like the person he was once. This can help in remembering him.

The funeral

The funeral is very important for you and other close relatives and friends, whatever your religious beliefs and those of the patient. What sort of ceremony would he have liked if he could have discussed it with you before the onset of the disease? It could be helpful to think this out long before his actual death. Thinking about the right end to his life and a ceremony to mark it can be the beginning of making more sense of his life and the beginning of the next stage of yours. Would he like flowers and music? Would he prefer a church service or a service in a crematorium? Would he have preferred to have had any religious observance at all or not? These are all very important questions and most of us are not sufficiently aware of the choices that we have. Registration of the death and cremation or burial of the body are obligatory, but beyond those formalities there are many options. You do not have to have any religious observance and can plan and organize your own ceremony in a crematorium with readings and music which are a reminder of the person as he was once. You can have a service in a church and cremation afterwards; but the committal can take place in the church and there is no need for anybody to go with the body to the crematorium. The ashes will be available later at the funeral director's. You must decide where you think the person would most have liked his ashes to be put. Where were your happiest times? These are all important decisions and ones which can help your understanding of the tragedy of his disease, disintegration and death. They can be stepping-stones along your own road to recovery and reintegration.

The funeral ceremony, wherever you choose to hold it, is an important time for you, your family and friends. It is a time when you can be brought back together again and it can become a precious memory. If it is at all possible those closest to you should eat together after the ceremony. It does not need to be an elaborate meal.

John's funeral was in a chapel in a cathedral which had become familiar to me. He had not known this chapel but would have loved it. There were many flowers which he would have enjoyed. His ashes were scattered from a pilot cutter in the North Sea where we had planned to spend time sailing during his retirement. There was a sharing in those last things which had been lacking in the last years of his life.

9 / Bereavement

Bereavement in Alzheimer's disease has started long before the death of the patient. It may have gone on for as long as ten years during his life before there is recognition that a bereavement is taking place and recovery from it can begin. Dementia is a disintegration of the whole person and such a disintegration can be felt by those closest to be a threat to their own integrity. Denial of the feelings aroused while caring for a dementing patient is normal, essential and necessary; but in time this threat of disintegration needs to be looked at and understood if the carer is to make a full recovery. Restoration to full health after bereavement is a normal process and usually occurs with the help of relatives and friends. But recovery after a death from Alzheimer's disease can take a very long time because of the nature of this long-lasting death.

Stages of grief

In 1970 Elizabeth Kubler-Ross wrote about the stages of grief. She described them as denial, anger, bargaining, depression and acceptance. Since then a number of other workers in the field of bereavement have described these stages in different ways. These include Colin Murray Parkes who in 1975 categorized the stages as those of alarm, searching, mitigation, anger and guilt and finally gaining a new identity. In 1978 Peter Speck described three stages of shock and disbelief, developing awareness, and resolution.

These descriptions can be useful for the bereaved person in seeing her feelings as normal, acceptable and understood. Descriptions of stages can be a help along the way and give the bereaved person some sense of others having experienced the same emotions. But I believe they can be unhelpful in providing some sort of check-list of normality to which she can feel that she is not measuring up. A bereaved person can feel abnormal if she has not accepted her grief within the average time. It can make her think 'I should try harder' or 'I ought to have accepted it by now.' There is also a danger that bereavement can become yet another modern disease or dis-ease which can be diagnosed, treated and become somebody else's responsibility. It can substitute for the bereaved person's need to actually experience it. Bereavement is as unique and individual as the number of people going through it. It can be as lonely as birth probably was and as death will be.

During the course of Alzheimer's disease bereavement has gone on for so long a time, and the threat to the carer's own personality has been so great, that recovery can also take a long time. All the 'should' ideas can be intellectually understandable but emotionally barren. The need for reconciliation and healing is of a much deeper significance than academic theories. It is all too easy to get caught up in the 'shoulds' and 'oughts' which can perpetuate the vicious circle of confusion, anger and despair.

However, on the plus side, because the disruption is so profound, recovery when it does come can be remarkable. I shall use here my own interpretation of the various stages of grief to show that bereavement after Alzheimer's disease will probably be complicated and prolonged. Prolonged grief has been called abnormal grief.

Abnormal grief

In one study of thirty-five people who had a breakdown after bereavement it was found that there were two common factors. One was a tendency for the grief to have been prolonged; and the other was for the reaction to bereavement to have been delayed. In this series the causes for the prolongation and delay were various. Bereavement after Alzheimer's disease must always incorporate these two 'at risk' factors; but, of course, this does not mean that everybody who has suffered such a bereavement will break down. In the group of people who had a breakdown there was much preoccupation with ideas of guilt and self-reproach. During the years that a carer has been looking after the patient with Alzheimer's disease she must suppress such ideas. She will have needed all her energy to cope with the constant demands of the dementing patient. Later the negative feelings may be very strong.

In prolonged and unresolvable grief, as occurs while being close to somebody with Alzheimer's disease, all previous experiences of bereavement, not necessarily from death and possibly going back to early childhood, may be reawakened. I felt at one point that bereavement after surviving a 'living' death from Alzheimer's disease had gone on for so long that full recovery for me would be impossible. Endurance of my own remaining life was all that I could reasonably expect.

Every loss in life, from infancy on, can be stirred and erupt and the pain become so great that it must be avoided and denied. The disintegration of a near person such as a spouse, a parent or a close friend can and does strike chords indicating our own lack of integrity. Each stage in the disintegration of the patient can cause a further threat to the integrity of the carer. The pain can cause disabling distress if it is acknowledged during the patient's life; but at a later date its recognition can be an opportunity for a new understanding of the self. There will be a remarkable opportunity not only for eventual recovery from bereavement but also for a new vision of the way in which the rest of the carer's life can be lived.

Shock and disbelief

These are described by Parkes as the first feelings after bereavement. Death in Alzheimer's disease is not sudden but a long drawn out process and for the carer the bereavement is gradual and prolonged. The sense of shock and disbelief may have manifested itself in the form of physical or mental distress over many years. Nobody outside can understand or believe what is happening between the dementing person and the spouse or near carer and the distress of the carer can be shown and more easily recognized in physical or mental illness. There may well be a withdrawal of both the patient and the carer from friends and relatives because of the inexplicable changes in both of them. This leads to increasing isolation. Eventually the patient escapes from the situation by death; but the carer will have a great deal of work and understanding to do if she wishes to rejoin life.

Change and loss

The whole process of loss in bereavement involves change. It means readjustment by the individual to the new situation in which she finds herself. Normally this time of adjustment and change will start after the death of the patient. However, during the time when the carer is looking after the dementing patient, she is already deeply involved in this change but is unaware of it. There is blindness to what is going on. This increases her sense of isolation and confusion because the real problem may remain hidden and secret.

A spouse, particularly a wife, will naturally cling to the relationship because of the loss of status in widowhood. Clinging to a relationship which is losing all meaning can be potentially destructive. It may be a sort of immunization against ever facing the facts of bereavement and 'real' widowhood when the partner finally dies. All sorts of strategies will have been developed for survival. My own sense of confusion about my identity, after I found myself on my own following my breakdown, was epitomized when I filled in a tax form. The options included 'divorced' and 'widowed'. I knew I was neither of those and finally chose 'separated'. I then realized that was not my official category so I added 'illegally'.

Feelings of guilt and anger

At the time of John's death and in the succeeding weeks there was some relief that his death had been peaceful, the family was together again and that for the last eighteen months of his life I had been able to play a small part in caring for him. A year later I was far more aware of all the many things that I had not been able to do to help him. I was acutely aware of all my inadequacies in our years together and of the futility of blaming his dementia for everything that had gone wrong in the last years of his life. All the 'if onlys' flooded in. I had great difficulty in forgiving myself that John's illness had occurred and also in forgiving John for all that I had suffered during his illness.

During the process of caring for somebody with dementia, there must be denial of feelings in order to cope with pressing day-to-day problems. Denial of feelings may have become a way of living and a strategy for survival. The anger and sense of outrage that this is happening can become inadmissible. Anger as a stage of bereavement is 'normal'; but if it has continued for many years while living with this chronic death, it can be too painful to admit or dare to recognize. The carer has not been rejected or abandoned just once by the death of the patient. She has been abandoned repeatedly over many years by the patient 'removing himself' from her and the relationship during his disintegration. It is an ongoing and potentially destructive anger, which may find an outlet as depression or physical illness. These can be temporary 'escape' routes, but in the end do not help resolve the bereavement and the recovery of the carer.

Longstanding denial of angry feelings and intense emotional pain can lead to an unrecognized resolution that 'I will not ever feel too much again. If I felt too much about anything it might hurt and I could not bear it. It might destroy me utterly.' This is a false sort of insurance against destruction. It may be a means of avoiding intense pain and anger but it will also prevent the experience of any joy, peace or love. It may appear safer but it is a sad way of readjusting and will be a constant deprivation that is self-inflicted.

The beginning of acceptance

By the second anniversary of John's death, the 'if onlys' were not as acute, but I still had a profound disquiet about my own inadequacies and a much greater awareness of my own need for help. I began to have some enthusiasm and hope that I could eventually become 'whole' again. Eventually I began to understand the inevitability of what had happened. I could then begin to accept John's illness and death as facts rather than reasons for my guilt and personal recrimination.

Naming things can make them more acceptable. If disintegration of a person can be called 'Alzheimer's disease' it makes it more bearable. It is known to be a disease that is unpreventable and incurable. There is nothing that you or anybody else could have done to stop it. The disease ran its course and the patient died. These are facts and can be distanced from your feelings of guilt. If total desolation can be named 'separation anxiety' or 'an abnormal grief pattern' it is also more bearable because it is more understandable. Some of the distress can then be shared by reading books about bereavement or obtaining help from a bereavement counsellor. These stages of acceptance can be useful, but eventually the theory and the process of naming must be integrated with emotional understanding.

The second part of acceptance can be the acceptance of your own personality, the way in which you have reacted to this long loss and an exploration of your own feelings and motives. The deeper understanding of oneself can be painful and many prefer to avoid it.

Recovery and renewal

During the long years of bereavement, loyalty to a disintegrating person and relationship, the strategies necessary for survival and coping can be in opposition to the sort of trusting, sharing and loving necessary for good physical, mental and emotional health. It is only through becoming open to the pain that real resolution of the grief can occur. It is probably now about sixteen years since the beginning of my own bereavement. Gradually, as I am able to accept all the pain and anger of those years, I am also able to feel again and assimilate some of the joy, the love and the fun of the relationship at its best. It has been easier to dwell on the loss and the futility than dare to feel the pain of the loss and then be able to recover the feelings of joy. The future can hold many surprises. I shall write more about emotional recovery, which is an essential part of physical recovery, in chapter 10.

Sources of help

People who can help

In 'normal' bereavement, family and friends will be the usual helpers. Professional helpers can include doctors, nurses, your minister of religion and bereavement counsellors. As you set the agenda for the care of the dementing patient, you must also be prepared to set an agenda for your own care. You must be honest about your own weakness and needs. You may have to ask for the help you do need; and you may have to reject help from somebody who is not helping you. At the same time as rejecting inappropriate help, you must be aware of your anger about your loss and the possibility that the anger is being thrown on to your helper.

Special help

If the grief is unbearable you may need temporary help in the form of tranquillizers or antidepressants. Your doctor will be able to prescribe these. They can be useful for short-term relief from the distress. The help of a psychiatrist can also be necessary.

Organizations

You may find help in organizations such as the Alzheimer's Disease Society or Cruse. A self-help group can be a valuable source of support, or you may find it too intrusive. You must be ready to accept what does help and reject what is unhelpful at any particular time.

Books and other writing

Choice of a helpful book will be very individual. There are many books about bereavement and some of them are given in the appendix.

The connection between the acceptance of pain and the resolution of grief with healing is beautifully expressed in *The Prophet* by Kahlil Gibran.

And a woman spoke, saying, Tell us of Pain.
And he said:
Your pain is the breaking of the shell that encloses your understanding.

Even as the stone of the fruit must break, that its heart may stand in the sun, so must you know pain.

And could you keep your heart in wonder at the daily miracles of your life, your pain would not seem less wondrous than your joy;

And you would accept the seasons of your heart, even as you have always accepted the seasons that pass over your fields.

And you would watch with serenity through the winters of your grief.

Much of your pain is self-chosen.

It is the bitter potion by which the physician within you heals your sick self.

Therefore trust the physician, and drink his remedy in silence and tranquillity:

For his hand, though heavy and hard, is guided by the tender hand of the Unseen.

And the cup he brings, though it burn your lips, has been fashioned of the clay which the Potter has moistened with his own sacred tears.

Bereavement during and after Alzheimer's disease has gone on for so long that it can have a profound and disruptive effect on the personality of the bereaved carer. However, if all the pain and losses can be accepted and understood there is an opportunity for change and for greater integrity of the personality of the carer during her remaining life. These changes can be the opposite to the disintegration that has happened to the patient during the latter years of his life and in which the carer has been so closely involved.

There can be a positive outcome if the connection between living with the person who disintegrates, and the threat to your own integrity, is faced and incorporated into the process of your own reintegration after bereavement.

First and second parts of life

It seems to me that in the twentieth-century developed world we are on the whole more effective at living the first half of our lives. During this period we are in the process of training our minds and bodies to achieve some sort of recognition. We are in the market for learning and for getting and keeping control of ourselves, our relationships and our surroundings. Perhaps it is also the time when we are filling, successfully or unsuccessfully, a series of roles. I shall write more about this under the heading of roles and role-playing (p. 94).

It can be the time of understanding life by what we have and not who we are. In Eric Fromm's book, *To Have or To Be*, there is an illuminating account of these two modes of living, with some explanation of the predominance of the 'having' mode in Western society. Some of our possessions such as our homes, cars, dogs and books are easily identifiable. My home, my husband and my children are easily recognizable to myself and those around and become extensions of myself. However, possessions can go beyond this to include my health, my illness or my problems. Having health or illness as some sort of possession is more easily understood than the state of being healthy or being sick in a society which is geared to the 'having' mode. A state of disintegration can be more easily accepted as 'having Alzheimer's disease'. Then the disease can become a recognizable if unwanted possession and at the same time be distanced from the person who has it. There is also the possibility of getting rid of the possession and the carer can then feel less threatened.

But for the majority of people the time comes, either rapidly or gradually, when the 'having' mode becomes irrelevant and most of their roles disappear. We can be left suspended between a dependent childhood, a long phase of role-playing and the prospect of old age and death. We may not realize what is happening. On the surface it is easier to try to carry on in the ways in which we have always lived our lives and deny that there is any change. The alternative is to stop, recognize and understand the profound changes that are occurring and consider alternative ways of living.

Disintegration could begin at the moment when we lose the opportunity to use our many roles, but fail to understand the significance of the loss. The loss of our main role of carer, when we are already battered by the experience of somebody else's disintegration, could be a similar moment. But it could also be an opportunity to look beyond the playing of roles and see it as a time to explore and develop our own hidden potential.

The second half of life, if we have accepted the 'having' mode unquestioningly, is a serial loss and deprivation with no possibility of gain. My health may go, and also my job and my money. My husband may die, my children leave home, my fertility can be taken away by a hysterectomy, and so on. During the time of approaching old age, many people do become poorer, give up professional status and power, move to smaller homes and even give up their car! We either give up all these possessions with good grace and possibly even with thankfulness, or hang on to them with ever-decreasing credibility and have them snatched from us while we protest. The loss of all of these can naturally lead to great sadness because we believed them to be necessary to our welfare.

Bereavement can be an opportunity for accepting a sort of 'mid-life' crisis. Most of us have spent the first fifty years or so of life entrenched in the 'having' mode, backed up by a culture favouring and supporting this mode. It is extremely difficult to accept all these losses as anything but failure. Only in a change of the person from the 'having' mode to the 'being' mode can such losses be understood as anything but bereavement. But the loss of the need for possessions can lead to a sort of liberation and eventually even to joy. It is a strange paradox that the acceptance of losses can lead to greater integration within the self; but hanging on to roles, images, possessions and all the outer trappings of life can lead to disintegration. Accepting the loss of spouse, home, financial security or professional role can also lead to a loss of fear and loss of anxiety about death. And this in turn leads to a strange sense of freedom and hope. What one still has at that point are the things within and they cannot be removed by any sort of material power.

I do not assume that the help that has been constructive for me will be equally so for the reader. I am sure that there are many ways of making this sort of discovery. The common factors will be the opportunity, the desire to change and daring to start. I do believe that for anybody trying to make sense of her own life after a bereavement from Alzheimer's disease there is the opportunity to look seriously and objectively at herself. Then, she can be in a position to make some realistic and clear-sighted choices about what is important to her and what she wants to do with the rest of her own life. All self-knowledge can be of immense value. Otherwise it is easy to drift into old age clinging to old habits, roles that are redundant, and a way of living that can be irrelevant and limiting. It can be a bit like trying to travel using a map which is out of date!

Roles and role-playing

There are going to be as many ways as there are people of making these changes and discoveries. A useful starting point for some may be to read Eric Berne's book *Games People Play*, which is an introduction to transactional analysis. He describes the archetypes within all of us of the parent, the child and the adult. These are the role models which are built into each of us and depend to some extent on our background and upbringing. Our use of them depends on the sort of real-life roles we achieve. The actual playing out of these can change from minute to minute in any particular encounter. In the course of one conversation I might change from using the role of parent to that of child, then into my adult role and back to parent again. The carer for the person with Alzheimer's disease can be forced into many and changing roles at bewildering speed. A dementing patient who still has control of the family's finances can be the most tyrannical of parents and the carer be the most dependent of children. On the other hand, as the patient's dementia and disintegration progress, the carer needs to assume the role of parent – and a fairly powerful one to cope with all the mess; but at the same time she may in reality be kept in the role of child and at a very dependent level.

In this switching of roles the archetype of the adult can be disintegrated and crushed between the competing archetypes of the parent and child. I had been blind to this problem during John's dementia and disintegration although it was most certainly there. I was too caught up in all the problems and my own emotional turmoil to see it. But I did become aware of it during my mother's disintegration.

At that time I saw and recognized the role of parent in her which had made her distant, authoritarian and unable to give me, her first child, the sort of mothering and tender love that could have made me feel secure as a baby. At the same time I saw that she was acting, during her period of disintegration and dependency, in the role of the child within her. The child was terrified of what would happen to her if she failed to be a good little girl. I saw that she had only managed to survive as an adult and reconcile these conflicting elements within herself by using my needs as a difficult baby with many health problems to satisfy her own needs for attention and support. The doctor who was presented with her child's problems could then assume the role of her parent. Suddenly, I became aware not only of the disturbance between the three archetypes in her but of the complexity of their reaction with those within me. I saw the screaming monster who had been me as a small child, and who still lurked within me, and the terrified child who was and still is my mother. The archetypes of the parent and the child had been exposed in my own understanding. I was better able to see both the parent role and the child role in both of us. And then gradually I became better able to accept and love both of them in both of us. In me the parent part had always been allowed to be public; but the child part had to remain hidden.

I have used this personal experience as an example of the way the use of roles can be understood; but, of course, it will not apply in precisely the same way to the reader. But perhaps for many of us a moment can present itself that can be used for greater understanding. Acceptance of some of our hidden and more secret inner selves can seem threatening but could mean greater integration. It might even prevent or lessen the possibility of disintegration.

Another book which might help the reader along the way of greater self-understanding is *The Road Less Travelled* by the American psychoanalyst M. Scott Peck.

Exploration of pain

My increased understanding of myself was not without pain. In caring for my mother it would have been easier and less painful for me to retreat into my role of doctor or powerful carer – or the parent role within me. That is the safer part of me and the more public part. It would have avoided much pain and that behaviour would have been normal and acceptable. The avoidance of pain is an important and acceptable fact of modern life and health care. Therapeutic drugs and anaesthetics screen us from many ills and horrifying physical and mental pain. We are all thankful that it is so. No longer is there a sense of moral outrage about the use of analgesia during childbirth, as there was before Queen Victoria used chloroform! We all have ways of finding instant, if passing, happiness, and most of these are socially acceptable. There are many ways of escaping from emotional pain and these include both physical and mental illness. These ideas are explored at length in *The Road Less Travelled*.

But, paradoxically, protecting ourselves from pain can limit our development as mature adults. It can also protect us from finding extraordinary joy. An exploration of those more hidden parts of ourselves, which can seem so unattractive and so necessary to keep secret, can be painful but reveal surprisingly good potential. During the process of living with a disintegrating person and after bereavement we can either resist any such understanding of ourselves or we can use the opportunity to explore some of those hidden depths.

Our outer and inner selves

Perhaps dementia and disintegration can occur in some people at a time when it is most difficult to keep the outer self and its roles and possessions of many sorts and the frail and secret inner self together. The roles that have kept some credibility for the person and for those around him have disappeared through changing status, changing age, poor physical health or even the threat of self-understanding. The break-up of the family unit and the children leaving home can be threats for a mother; promotion or retirement of the spouse can threaten a husband or wife. The world of outer reality is the normal one for us in the Western world during most of our lives. It is the life of the body and the mind, of material possessions, recognizable roles and material succes or failure. If the outer reality has always been all-important, then changes within it may be overpowering for somebody with a poor sense of their own inner reality.

As an example of the possibility of developing our sense of an inner reality instead of clinging to an outer reality which is changing or gone, I shall describe a recent walk that I took. I was writing this book sitting at my word processor in a small city-centre terrace house. It was surprisingly hot weather and I kept thinking of all sorts of other activities that would be much more pleasant than sitting and trying to pin down my thoughts. Eventually, I decided to go and deliver a birthday card I had forgotten to post. I decided to take a short cut through a small park created from a bomb site. I realized with some surprise that it was three years since I had walked that way. I used to walk there frequently when I had a dog but she died just a month after my husband's death.

It was a great relief to find such a good excuse to escape from the discipline of writing. The ground was white with daisies and punctuated with the gold spots of dandelions. At the end of the park there used to be a small children's playground with swings, roundabout, seesaw and climbing frame. I discovered that it had disappeared and I experienced a sensation of loss. I stood there and remembered the day almost exactly seven years ago when I had moved into my house and the crazy late-night end to that day. The cousin who had helped me with the move, and who is now dead, his wife and I had bought fish and chips, and walked through the park eating them in a late evening mist. We then spent a ridiculously happy hour playing on all the children's equipment. I stood there seeing and feeling every moment of that brief time. The swings and roundabouts had gone, my cousin is dead, my dog is dead and John, who was not physically with us, is also dead. I remembered many other losses and sadnesses and much pain. However, my feeling of joy in the memory of that extraordinary hour was totally alive and real to me. I could even think of John with us and also enjoying the hour and I realized that those joyful memories can be recalled at any time. Perhaps that inner reality is now more important for me than the external realities which have changed and gone.

So much of our inner selves is made up of all the throwaway events, facts and feelings for which we have had no space in our busy lives. Some of them have been thrown away because they were painful or seemed irrelevant. But the thoughts and feelings continue to lie around somewhere inside us. We all know some version of the saying that 'inside every psychiatrist is a nutter' or 'inside every policeman is a criminal'. And the comment made in a tone of considerable surprise, 'I never thought she had it in her!' Inside, the upright, pious and responsible carer may be a sexy bombshell or a demon explorer. The part of us that we keep hidden can be surprisingly powerful, very interesting and a source of new strength. Here is an Indian story which illustrates what I am trying to explain.

Each day the king sat in state hearing petitions and dispensing justice. Each day a holy man, dressed in the robe of an ascetic beggar, approached the king and without a word offered him a piece of very ripe fruit. Each day the king accepted the 'present' from the beggar and without a thought handed it to his treasurer who stood behind the throne. Each day the beggar, again without a word, withdrew and vanished into the crowd.

Year after year this precise same ritual occurred every day the king sat in office. Then one day, some ten years after the holy man first appeared, something different happened. A tame monkey, having escaped from the women's apartments in the inner palace, came bounding into the hall and leaped up on to the arm of the king's throne. The ascetic beggar had just presented the king with his usual gift of fruit, but this time instead of passing it on to his treasurer as was his usual custom, the king handed it over to his monkey. When the animal bit into it, a precious jewel dropped out and fell to the floor.

The king was amazed and quickly turned to his treasurer behind him. 'What has become of all the others?' he asked. But the treasurer had no answer. Over all the years he had simply thrown the unimpressive 'gifts' through a small upper window in the treasure house, not even bothering to unlock the door. So he excused himself and ran quickly to the vault. He opened it and hurried to the area beneath the little window. There, on the floor, lay a mass of rotten fruit in various stages of decay.

But amidst the garbage of many years lay a heap of precious gems.

Contemplation

We shall each find a different way of developing a greater awareness of our own inner selves if we choose to do so. The individual way will depend on our own background, upbringing and culture. Essentially it could be described as awareness of the spiritual part of us. For some it can be by the way of contemplation or meditation. There are many ways of practising contemplation either individually or as part of a group. You may want to investigate some of these for yourself. There are numerous books on the subject and one that I have found particularly helpful is *Sadhana A Way to God* by Anthony de Mello. It is sub-titled 'Christian Exercises In Eastern Form' and is described as a 'how-to-do-it book . . . a series of spiritual exercises for entering the contemplative state, blending psychology, spiritual therapy and practices of both Eastern and Western traditions'. Here is an exercise from this book which you may find helpful.

Close your eyes once again. Get in touch with sensations in various parts of your body.

The ideal would be not even to think of the various parts of your body as 'hands' or 'legs' or 'back' but just to move from one sensation to another and give no labels or names to your limbs and organs as you sense them.

If you notice an urge to move or shift your position, do not give in to it. Just become aware of the urge and the bodily discomfort, if any, that gives rise to the urge.

Stay with the exercise for a few minutes. You will gradually feel a certain stillness in your body. Do not explicitly rest in the stillness. Go on with your awareness exercise and leave the stillness to take care of itself.

If you become distracted, get back to the awareness of body sensations, moving from one to another, until your body becomes still once again and your mind quietens with your body and you are able to sense once again this stillness that brings peace and a foretaste of contemplation and of God. However, I repeat, do not explicitly rest in the stillness.

The moment when we first see clearly a glimpse of our own death can either be the moment of a frenetic escape into a dwindling outer reality or another opportunity of self-knowledge. We can either rush into any number of escape routes as we look at a long vista of helplessness and hopelessness. Or we can begin to do things like learn active stillness and start to explore our inner selves.

Story-telling

The events that have occurred are never the same as the story about those events; and there may be many different stories connected with the same events. The difference can be as great as the news of a gale in the shipping forecast and a true story of shipwreck and rescue that happened during the same gale. Events are facts but the story contains both the facts and also the meaning behind them for the person who has lived at the centre. It can be useful to see one's own life as a personal story. By understanding the story of one's life it can be more easily seen as a whole. Life is always a series of events but the interpretation and editing of them is what brings meaning to that person's life.

For example, I recently had a long wait at Heathrow airport to meet some of my family. I spent the time in the coffee bar at Terminal 3 filling in a survey form about my own medical career.

It was a piece of research on what happens to medical women graduates. I nearly abandoned it after the first two questions because my career was such a sorry tale of failure and incompleteness. Near the end was a question, 'If you are not working now are you actively seeking work?' At that point I stopped and surveyed the story of my medical career. I realized that there was an extraordinary disparity between my failure as seen from the point of view of the academic researcher looking at women in medicine and my own remarkable survival, having practised many sorts of medicine in many places. This was my story and there was a big difference between the facts entered on the survey form and later no doubt on a computer and the meaning behind them for me. I was a failed doctor but a maturing person. My story was very individual and could not be written on a survey form.

My elderly mother, when her mind was very frail, was persuaded to write her memoirs. She had not done any writing since she was at school, apart from many letters and writing her diary. She has written and is still editing a remarkable story which is proving of immense interest to the whole family. It is full of most interesting stories about members of our family. She keeps saying, 'But I thought all that was so boring and none of your would be interested.' Of course it is not boring. This is a part of our story and it helps to make more sense of all our lives. What she saw as failure and things which were not nice to make public are fascinating insights into ways in which members of the family have behaved over several generations. She has not only made more sense of her own life but has become the family's historian and her book will long be handed down and treasured.

Any society will have some common history and possibly religion; but it will have many individual stories which can be woven together. In Samoa, the old people and particularly the women are the story-tellers. They can remember the past of the families, the village communities and the tribes. These stories are told and retold to the coming generations. This gives the old people in Samoa a special place of importance in their communities. In the same way, my mother has assumed a new importance as the family story-teller. I believe that this art of story-telling, which our modern communications have helped to destroy, needs to be restored to a place of importance in our culture. The listener and the watcher with radio and television are passive. They do not have the opportunity to ask, argue and talk back; and an essential role of an old person has been lost.

The facts of our lives do not change; but the story of our lives will as we attach different meaning to those facts and become more in touch with our inner selves. Here is an exercise which you may find useful, taken from Gerard Hughes' book *God of Surprises*:

Write your own obituary notice. This may seem an odd and morbid suggestion, but try it first before deciding it is a waste of time. Do not write the obituary which you are afraid you might have, but the kind of obituary which, in your wildest dreams, you would love to have. Do not analyse it, or try to think it out too clearly, but allow your fancy to run free. Having once done it, return to it now and again and see if you want to add to it or correct it.

This can be a very useful exercise for getting more in touch with your inner life, above all with your desires which, as we shall see later, are at the core of our inner lives and to determine their direction.

As children, we all wanted to know what the end of the story was and this is a chance of finding out; but there is the added bonus that while we are still alive the meaning of our lives and the ending of them is still open to change.

The person who has Alzheimer's disease probably could never

have written the story of his life or understood its meaning; but the carer having shared the patient's disintegration may ultimately be in a position to understand more profoundly the meaning of her own life.

Appendix 1

Useful books

The Poison that Waits? The script of a *Horizon* programme obtainable from the B B C, P O Box 7, London, W3 6XJ. Cheque or postal order for £1.75 payable to Broadcasting Support Services.

'Regular Review' Recent research on the causes of Alzheimer's disease in the *British Medical Journal*, 297, 1988, 807–10.

The 36-Hour Day by N. Mace and P. Robins, Hodder and Stoughton in conjunction with Age Concern, 1985.

Dementia and Mental Illness in the Old by Elaine Murphy, Papermac, 1986.

Alzheimer's Disease and Related Disorders ed. M. Roth and L. L. Iversen, British Medical Bulletin published for the British Council, Churchill Livingstone, 1986.

Alzheimer's Disease: Coping with a Living Death by Robert T. Woods, Souvenir Press, 1989.

Caring for the Alzheimer Patient – a Practical Guide ed. Raye Lynne Dippel and J. Thomas Hutton, Prometheus Books, 1984.

Appendix 2

Useful addresses

Age Concern England
60 Pitcairn Road, Mitcham, Surrey CR4 3LL.
Tel: 01–640 5431.

Age Concern (Scotland)
33 Castle Street, Edinburgh.
Tel: 031–225 5000.

Alzheimer's Disease Society
158/160 Balham High Road, London SW12 9BN.
Tel: 01–675 6557/8/9/0.

Alzheimer's Disease Society in Scotland
3rd Floor, 40 Shandwick Place, Edinburgh EH2 4RT.
Tel: 031–225 1453.

Association of Crossroads Care
94 Coton Road, Warwickshire CV21 4LN.
Tel: 0788–73653.

British Red Cross Society
9 Grosvenor Crescent, London SW1X 7EJ.
Tel: 01–235 5454.

Carers' National Association
29 Chilworth Mews, London W2 3RG.
Tel: 01–724 7776.

Citizens Advice Bureaux
see your local telephone directory.

Court of Protection
25 Store Street, London WC1E 7BP.
Tel: 01–636 6877.

Cruse
Cruse House, 126 Sheen Road, Richmond, Surrey TW9 1UR.
Tel: 01–940 4818/9047.

Disablement Income Group
Attlee House, 28 Commercial Street, London E1 6LR.
Tel: 01–247 2128/6877.

Distressed Gentlefolk's Aid Association
Vicarage Gate House, Vicarage Gate, London W8 4AQ.
Tel: 01–229 9341.

Help the Aged
16/18 St James' Walk, London EC1R 0BE.
Tel: 01–253 0253.

Independent Living Fund, PO Box 183, Nottingham NG8 3RD.

Law Society
113 Chancery Lane, London WC1.

Local Health Councils
see under Health Services in your local telephone directory.

MIND
22 Harley Street, London W1N 2ED.
Tel: 01–637 0741.

RADAR (The Royal Association for Disability and Rehabilitation) 25 Mortimer Street, London W1N 8AB.
Tel: 01–637 5400.

Samaritans
see your local telephone directory.

Social Services Department
see your local telephone directory.

Index

abnormalities, 28, 44
  see also brain changes; chromosome 21; Down's syndrome
absentmindedness, 36
  see also memory
acetylcholine, 32–3
acute infective illnesses, 34
Age Concern, 66, 70–1, 105–6
ageing, 36–7, 61
AIDCALL alarm, 70
AIDS, 35
alcohol abuse, 53
aluminium, 26, 29–33
Alzheimer, Alois, 21
Alzheimer's disease
  causes, 25–6
  commonest type of dementia, 21
  definition, 22–3
  diagnosis, 2, 5, 6–7, 19, 46, 49, 51–3, 56, 61, 65
  genetic factors, 25–9
  infective agents, 29
  management, 2, 45–7, 51–2, 56–63, 65, 68, 74
  onset, 24–5, 34, 36, 41, 46, 75
  untreatable condition, 14, 44–6, 49, 87
  see also acetylcholine; aluminium; bereavement; brain changes; *British Medical Journal*; death; dementia; depression; Forsythe, John; *Horizon*; neurofibrillary tangles; professional help

Alzheimer's Disease Society, 26–7, 37, 66, 69–70, 89, 106
amyloid proteins, 28
anaemia, 54–5
anger, 27, 38, 54, 58, 61, 72, 82, 86–9
  see also bereavement; depression
antiobiotics, 34, 78
Association of Crossroads Care, 106
autosomal dominant genetic disease, 27

behaviour, 11–12, 26, 36, 41, 45–8, 69
  see also personality changes
bereavement
  abnormal grief, 83–4, 88
  acceptance, 87–8, 90
  Alzheimer's disease as 'ongoing' bereavement, 77, 82–3, 91
  anger as a stage of, 86–7
  counselling, 89
  life after, 91–104
  process of, 57–8, 71, 85
  recovery from, 19, 83, 85, 87–8
  shock and disbelief, 85
  use of tranquillizers and antidepressants, 89
  writings about, 89–90, 92, 99–103
  see also professional help; religious writings; Samoa; voluntary organizations
Berne, Eric
  Games People Play, 94